Take Control of COPD

A Doctor's Practical Guide to Better Breathing

Dr Prabhat Das

MD, PhD, FACP

Better Health with Dr Das Series

Hardcover ISBN: 978-1-971672-43-4

Paperback ISBN: 978-1-971672-42-7

eBook ISBN: 978-1-971672-41-0

Printed in the United States of America

Disclaimer

This book is intended solely for educational and informational purposes. It is not meant to replace personal medical advice, diagnosis, or treatment.

Although I am a licensed physician, reading this book does not establish a doctor-patient relationship. Each individual's health condition, medical history, and risk factors are unique. Any medical decision should be made in partnership with your own healthcare professional who understands your specific situation.

Medical science is continually advancing. New research and updated guidelines may lead to changes in recommendations over time.

About the Author

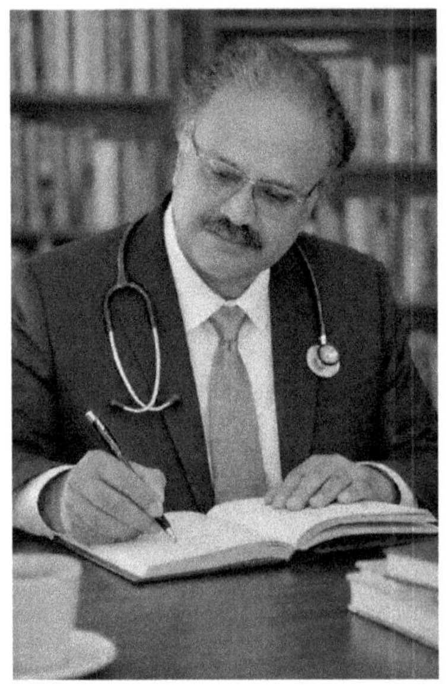

I am Dr Prabhat Das, MD, PhD, FACP. My journey in medicine began in India and, over the past thirty-five years, has continued in the United States, where I have had the privilege of caring for patients across a wide range of medical settings. I am trained in Internal Medicine, Pulmonary Diseases, and Critical Care. For me, medicine has never been just a profession. It has been a lifelong commitment shaped by learning, service, and a deep respect for the trust patients place in their physician.

Over the years, I have had the honor of caring for patients in many different situations. I have seen individuals in my office for routine concerns, treated urgent conditions in busy emergency rooms, managed serious illnesses in the hospital, and cared for critically ill patients in intensive care units. Each setting has taught me something valuable. Each patient has added to my understanding of what it truly means to care for another human being.

But one lesson has stood above all others. Medicine is not only about tests, diagnoses, or treatments. It is about people. It is about listening carefully, understanding fears that are often left unspoken, and guiding patients through uncertainty with clarity and compassion. Again and again, I have seen that what people want most is simple, trustworthy information. They want to understand what is happening in their bodies. They want to feel confident about the decisions they are making for their health and for their families.

These experiences have deeply shaped how I think about health, illness, prevention, and the human side of healing.

That is the reason behind the '**Better Health with Dr Das Series'**. Through these books, I hope to reach individuals I may never meet in person but who are searching for clear and reliable guidance. In today's world, health information is everywhere, yet much of it is confusing, overwhelming, and sometimes misleading. My goal is to cut through that noise and present important medical topics in a way that is simple, practical, and reassuring.

Every page of this series is guided by two foundations: reliable scientific knowledge and decades of real-world clinical experience. I want you, the reader, to feel informed, confident, and empowered. Not overwhelmed. Not confused. But clear about what you can do, step by step, to improve your health.

If even one reader feels less anxious, more informed, or better prepared to take control of their health after reading these books, then this work has served its purpose.

Helping people live healthier, longer, more confident and better-informed lives remains one of the greatest privileges of my life.

TABLE OF CONTENTS:

CHAPTER 1: Understanding COPD – The Big Picture

What This Book Is Really About

Over the years, I have met many patients who come to me with a quiet worry.

"Doctor, I get breathless. Is something seriously wrong?"

Sometimes they have already been told they have COPD. Sometimes they have never heard the term before.

But almost all of them share one thing.

Uncertainty.

This book is written to remove that uncertainty.

I am not writing this as a textbook. I am writing this the way I explain things to my own patients, sitting across from me in my office, trying to understand what is happening to their body.

By the end of this book, my goal is simple.

You should understand your condition clearly, feel more in control, and know exactly what you can do to live better.

What Is COPD in Simple Terms

COPD stands for Chronic Obstructive Pulmonary Disease.

That sounds complicated, but the idea is actually quite simple.

Chronic means long-term

Obstructive means something is blocking airflow

Pulmonary refers to the lungs

So COPD is a long-term condition where airflow in the lungs is partially blocked.

This makes it harder to breathe, especially when you try to exhale.

Patients often describe it in very practical ways:

"I feel like I cannot get the air out."
"I get tired quickly when I walk."
"I have to stop to catch my breath."

These are not just symptoms. They are signals from your lungs.

Why Breathing Becomes Difficult

To understand COPD, it helps to visualize how normal breathing works.

When you breathe in, air travels through your airways into tiny air sacs in the lungs. These air sacs exchange oxygen and carbon dioxide.

When you breathe out, the used air leaves easily.

In COPD, two main problems develop:

The airways become narrowed and inflamed

The air sacs lose their elasticity

Because of this:

Air gets trapped inside the lungs

It becomes difficult to push air out

Fresh air cannot enter efficiently

This leads to that familiar feeling of breathlessness.

The Two Main Types of COPD

COPD is not a single disease. It is a combination of two conditions.

Chronic Bronchitis

This involves:

Long-term inflammation of the airways

Persistent cough

Increased mucus production

Patients often say:
"I always have phlegm. It never really goes away."

Emphysema

This affects the air sacs.

The walls of the air sacs are damaged

They lose their elasticity

Oxygen exchange becomes less efficient

Patients may not cough much, but they feel breathless with activity.

Most patients have a combination of both.

Why COPD Develops Slowly

One important thing to understand is this.

COPD does not happen overnight.

It develops gradually over many years.

During this time:

Damage builds up slowly

Symptoms remain mild at first

The body adapts

Many patients ignore early symptoms because they seem minor.

"I just get a little tired."
"I am just getting older."

By the time symptoms become noticeable, the disease is already established.

Why Early Understanding Matters

This is where knowledge becomes powerful.

If you understand COPD early:

You can slow its progression

You can prevent complications

You can maintain a better quality of life

If ignored:

Symptoms worsen gradually

Daily activities become harder

Independence may be affected

The difference lies in awareness and timely action.

How Common Is COPD

COPD is one of the most common chronic diseases worldwide.

In the United States:

Millions of people are living with COPD

Many more remain undiagnosed

It is especially common in people over the age of 40, but it can occur earlier in some cases.

The important point is this.

You are not alone.

What Is COPD?

CHRONIC BRONCHITIS
EMPHYSEMA
Narrowed Airway
Air Trapping
Normal Lung
Open Airway
Inflamed & Mucus
Damaged Alveoli
Chronic Cough & Mucus
• Loss of Alveoli Elasticity
• Trapped Air

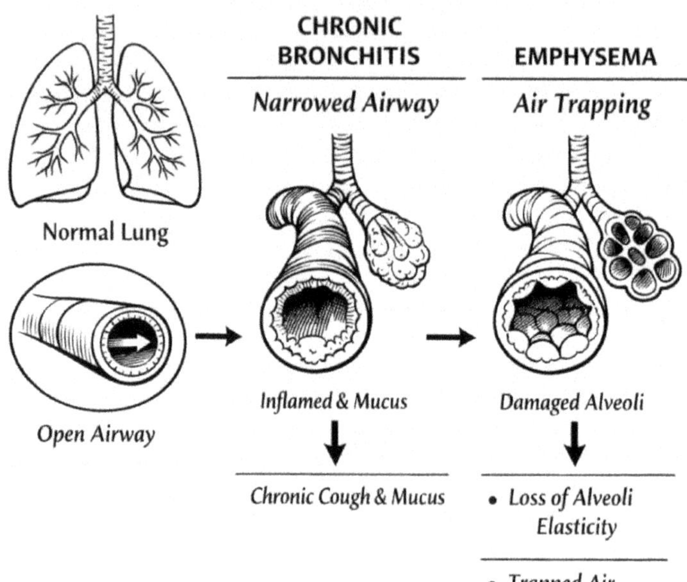

Why COPD Is Often Misunderstood

Despite being common, COPD is often misunderstood.

Some believe:

It happens only to smokers

Nothing can be done about it

Breathlessness is normal with age

All of these are incorrect.

These misconceptions delay diagnosis and treatment.

One of the main goals of this book is to correct these misunderstandings.

A Patient Story That Stays with Me

I remember a patient who came to see me after years of ignoring his symptoms.

He said:
"Doctor, I thought it was just aging. I never imagined it could be something serious."

We evaluated him and found clear signs of COPD.

The good news was that even at that stage, we could help him.

With treatment, lifestyle changes, and regular follow-up:

His symptoms improved

He became more active

His confidence returned

This is a pattern I have seen many times.

Understanding leads to action. Action leads to improvement.

What This Means for You

If you are reading this, you are already taking the most important step.

You are trying to understand.

COPD may be a chronic condition, but it is manageable.

With the right approach:

You can breathe better

You can stay active

You can maintain independence

This journey begins with knowledge.

Chapter Summary

COPD is a long-term condition that limits airflow in the lungs

It develops gradually over many years

The two main components are chronic bronchitis and emphysema

Breathlessness occurs due to airflow limitation and air trapping

Early symptoms are often ignored or misunderstood

COPD is common but frequently underdiagnosed

Understanding the condition early helps improve outcomes

Action Plan for You

Take your symptoms seriously
Do not ignore breathlessness or persistent cough

Seek proper evaluation
Early diagnosis makes a difference

Begin learning about your condition
Knowledge gives you control

Stay open to treatment and lifestyle changes
Small steps can lead to meaningful improvement

Transition to Next Chapter

Now that you understand what COPD is, the next important question is this: Why does it happen? In the next chapter, we will explore the causes and risk factors, so you can understand what led to this condition and how to prevent further damage.

CHAPTER 2: Why COPD Happens – Causes and Risk Factors

Understanding the "Why" Behind the Disease

After hearing the diagnosis of COPD, one of the first questions patients ask me is:

"Doctor, how did this happen to me?"

It is a very important question.

Because when you understand the cause, you begin to understand what you can change, what you cannot, and what steps you must take next.

COPD does not develop randomly. There are clear reasons behind it. In most cases, it is the result of long-term exposure to harmful substances that damage the lungs gradually.

Let us look at these causes in a simple and practical way.

Smoking – The Most Important Cause

There is no way to discuss COPD honestly without talking about smoking.

Smoking is the leading cause of COPD.

Cigarette smoke contains thousands of chemicals. Many of them are toxic to the lungs.

Over time, smoking:

Irritates the airways

Causes chronic inflammation

Damages the air sacs

Reduces the lungs' ability to repair themselves

This damage builds slowly over years.

Not everyone who smokes develops COPD, but the risk is very high.

And the longer and heavier the smoking history, the greater the damage.

Secondhand Smoke – A Hidden Risk

Even if you do not smoke, exposure to smoke from others can harm your lungs.

Living with a smoker or working in environments where smoking is common can lead to:

Chronic airway irritation

Increased risk of lung disease

Many patients are surprised when they learn this.

They say, "But I never smoked."

And yet, their lungs have been exposed for years.

Indoor Air Pollution -An Often Overlooked Cause

In many parts of the world, indoor pollution is a major cause of COPD.

This includes:

Smoke from cooking fuels such as wood or coal

Poorly ventilated kitchens

Burning of biomass fuels

Long-term exposure to these conditions can damage the lungs in a similar way to smoking.

Even in developed countries, exposure to indoor pollutants can occur in certain settings.

Occupational Exposure – What You Breathe at Work Matters

Your workplace can have a significant impact on your lung health.

Jobs involving exposure to:

Dust

Chemical fumes

Industrial gases

increase the risk of COPD.

Examples include:

Construction work

Mining

Factory work

Agriculture

Many patients do not connect their work environment with their symptoms.

But years of exposure can leave a lasting impact.

Environmental Pollution – The Air Around You

Air pollution is another contributing factor.

Living in areas with:

High traffic pollution

Industrial emissions

Poor air quality

can increase the risk of lung damage.

While this may not be the sole cause, it adds to the overall burden on the lungs.

Causes and Risk Factors for COPD

COPD usually happens when the lungs are exposed to harmful particles or gases for many years. Here are the main causes and risk factors.

MAIN CAUSES

SMOKING
The Leading Cause

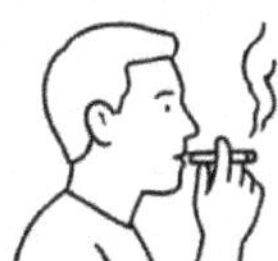

Cigarette smoke damages the airways and air sacs in the lungs.

SECONDHAND SMOKE
Still Harmful

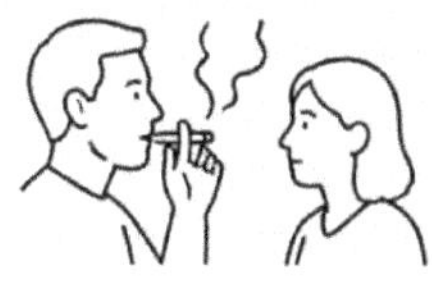

Breathing smoke from others can also increase risk.

LONG-TERM EXPOSURE TO AIR POLLUTION
Outdoors and Indoors

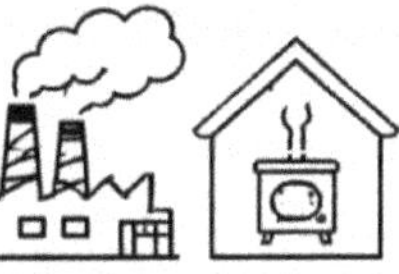

Polluted air and cooking or heating with solid fuels can harm the lungs.

OTHER IMPORTANT RISK FACTORS

OCCUPATIONAL DUST AND CHEMICALS

Dust, fumes, and chemicals at work can damage lungs over time.

GENETICS
(Alpha-1 Antitrypsin Deficiency)

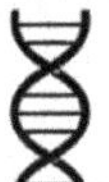

A rare inherited condition that can lead to COPD, especially in non-smokers.

CHRONIC LUNG INFECTIONS IN CHILDHOOD

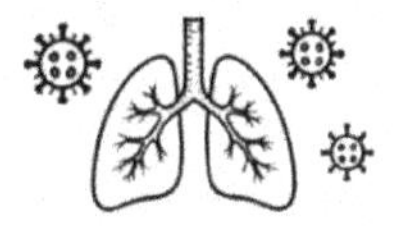

Repeated lung infections may affect lung growth and increase risk later.

AGING

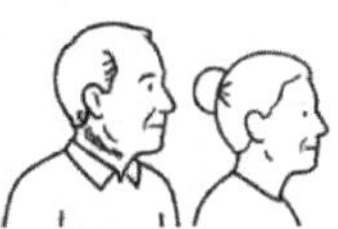

Lung function naturally declines with age, which can add to the risk.

ASTHMA HISTORY

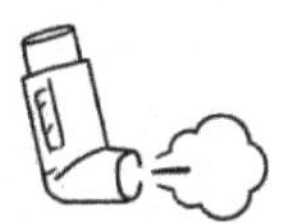

People with asthma may have a higher chance of developing COPD.

POOR LUNG GROWTH

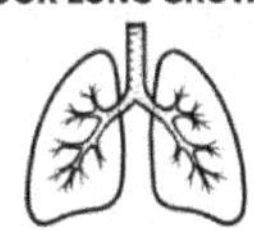

Lungs that did not fully develop can lead to lower lung reserve and higher risk.

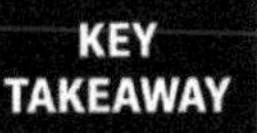

Smoking is the biggest cause of COPD, but other factors like pollution, work exposures, genetics, and lung infections also play a role.

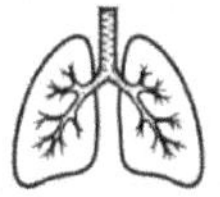

Genetic Factors – When Risk Is Inherited

In some cases, COPD develops due to genetic reasons.

The most well-known condition is **alpha-1 antitrypsin deficiency**.

This is a rare inherited disorder where the lungs are more vulnerable to damage.

Patients with this condition:

May develop COPD at a younger age

May have little or no smoking history

Recognizing this condition is important because it can influence both treatment and family screening.

Childhood Lung Development – The Early Years Matter

Your lung health in adulthood is influenced by your early years.

Factors such as:

Frequent childhood respiratory infections

Poor nutrition

Exposure to smoke in early life

can affect lung development.

If the lungs do not develop fully, they are more vulnerable later in life.

This is an area that many people overlook.

Repeated Infections – A Contributing Factor

Frequent respiratory infections over time can also contribute to lung damage.

Each infection:

Causes inflammation

Weakens the airways

Reduces lung function

Over years, this repeated injury can add up.

Why Some People Develop COPD and Others Do Not

This is a question I hear often.

“Doctor, I know people who smoked more than I did, but they are fine. Why me?”

The answer is that COPD is influenced by multiple factors.

These include:

Duration and intensity of exposure

Genetic susceptibility

Overall health

Environmental factors

Each person's lungs respond differently.

So while exposure is important, individual susceptibility also plays a role.

The Role of Aging

As we age:

Lung function naturally declines slightly

The ability to repair damage decreases

This makes older adults more vulnerable to the effects of long-term exposure.

However, aging alone does not cause COPD.

It works together with other risk factors.

A Practical Example

I remember two patients with similar smoking histories.

One developed severe COPD. The other had only mild symptoms.

The difference was not just smoking.

One had additional exposure to dust at work and had frequent infections in childhood.

This combination increased his risk.

This example highlights an important point.

COPD is usually the result of multiple factors acting together.

Why This Knowledge Is Important for You

Understanding the cause of your COPD helps you in two ways.

First, it helps you accept the condition with clarity rather than confusion.

Second, and more importantly, it helps you prevent further damage.

For example:

If smoking is the cause, quitting becomes essential

If exposure is the issue, reducing it becomes a priority

You may not be able to change the past.

But you can definitely influence your future.

Chapter Summary

COPD develops due to long-term damage to the lungs

Smoking is the leading cause

Secondhand smoke also increases risk

Indoor pollution and occupational exposure are important factors

Environmental pollution contributes to lung damage

Genetic conditions can play a role

Childhood lung health influences adult risk

Repeated infections may contribute to disease development

COPD usually results from multiple factors combined

Action Plan for You

Identify your risk factors
Understand what may have contributed to your condition

Eliminate ongoing exposure
Stop smoking and avoid harmful environments

Protect your lungs moving forward
Every step now helps prevent further damage

Discuss family history if relevant
Especially in early-onset cases

Focus on what you can control
Your future lung health depends on your current actions

Transition to Next Chapter

Now that you understand why COPD develops, the next important step is recognizing its symptoms. In the next chapter, we will look closely at the signs and symptoms of

COPD, so you can identify them early and respond appropriately.

CHAPTER 3: Recognizing the Symptoms – Listening to Your Body

Why Symptoms Are Often Missed

One of the most striking things I have seen in my practice is this.

Many patients live with symptoms for years without realizing something is wrong.

They say:

“I thought it was just aging.”

“I assumed I was out of shape.”

“It did not seem serious at first.”

And that is exactly how COPD behaves.

It begins quietly. Slowly. Almost unnoticed.

By the time symptoms become obvious, the disease has already progressed.

That is why learning to recognize early symptoms is so important.

Shortness of Breath – The Most Common Symptom

If there is one symptom that defines COPD, it is breathlessness.

At first, it appears only during activity:

Climbing stairs

Walking uphill

Carrying groceries

Later, it may occur even with simple tasks:

Walking on level ground

Getting dressed

Talking while moving

In advanced stages, some patients feel breathless even at rest.

Patients often describe it in their own words:

"I get winded easily."

"I cannot keep up with others."

"I have to stop and catch my breath."

These descriptions are very important.

They reflect how COPD affects daily life.

Common Symptoms of COPD

COPD can cause a *rarge* of symptoms that may gradually worsen over time. Here are five of the most common ones:

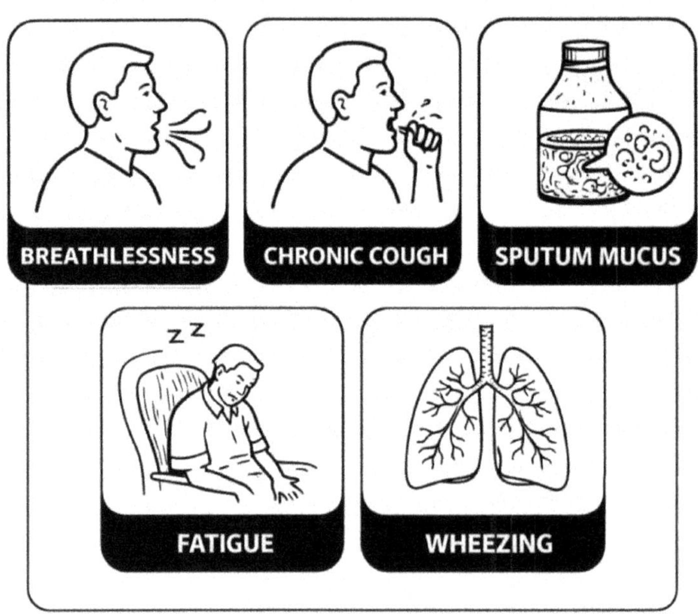

Chronic Cough – Often Ignored

A persistent cough is another key symptom.

It may:

Be present most days

Last for months or years

Be worse in the morning

Many patients dismiss it, especially if they smoke.

They call it a "smoker's cough."

But a chronic cough is not normal.

It is a sign that the airways are irritated and inflamed.

Sputum Production – What It Tells You

Along with cough, many patients produce mucus, also called sputum.

This may be:

Clear

White

Yellow or green during infections

Some patients say:
"I always have to clear my throat."
"I bring up phlegm every morning."

This is typical of chronic bronchitis.

Changes in sputum can also signal a flare-up.

Fatigue – The Silent Symptom

Fatigue is often overlooked.

Breathing in COPD requires more effort.

This constant effort:

Uses more energy

Leads to tiredness

Patients may feel:

Low energy

Reduced stamina

Difficulty completing daily tasks

They may not connect this to their lungs.

But it is an important part of the disease.

Wheezing – A Whistling Sound

Some patients experience wheezing.

This is a whistling or musical sound during breathing.

It occurs because:

Air is passing through narrowed airways

Not all patients have wheezing, but when present, it is a useful clue.

Chest Tightness – A Feeling of Pressure

Some patients describe a sensation of tightness in the chest.

It may feel like:

Pressure

Constriction

Difficulty expanding the chest fully

This symptom varies from person to person.

Frequent Respiratory Infections

Patients with COPD often have repeated infections.

These may include:

Colds

Bronchitis

Pneumonia

Each infection can:

Worsen symptoms

Delay recovery

Lead to flare-ups

Frequent infections are an important warning sign.

Subtle Early Signs You Should Not Ignore

Early symptoms are often mild.

They may include:

Slight decrease in stamina

Occasional breathlessness

Mild cough

Because these symptoms develop gradually, patients adjust their lifestyle without realizing it.

They may:

Avoid stairs

Walk slower

Reduce activity

This adaptation hides the progression of the disease.

How Symptoms Progress Over Time

COPD symptoms usually follow a gradual pattern.

Early Stage:

Mild breathlessness during activity

Occasional cough

Moderate Stage:

More noticeable breathlessness

Regular cough and sputum

Advanced Stage:

Breathlessness with minimal activity

Frequent flare-ups

Reduced independence

Understanding this progression helps you recognize where you stand.

Why Patients Delay Seeking Help

There are several reasons why patients do not seek care early:

Symptoms seem mild

They attribute it to aging

They do not want to "overreact"

Lack of awareness

Unfortunately, this delay allows the disease to progress.

A Practical Example

I remember a patient who said:

"Doctor, I stopped climbing stairs years ago. I did not think much of it."

When we discussed further, it became clear that he had gradually reduced his activity to avoid breathlessness.

His body had adapted. But the disease had progressed.

This is very common.

When Should You Seek Medical Attention

You should not wait for severe symptoms.

Seek evaluation if you have:

Persistent breathlessness

Chronic cough

Regular sputum production

Reduced ability to perform daily activities

Early evaluation leads to better outcomes.

Listening to Your Body

Your body gives signals.

The problem is not that symptoms are absent.

The problem is that they are often ignored.

Learning to listen to your body is one of the most important steps in managing COPD.

What This Means for You

If you recognize these symptoms in yourself:

Do not ignore them.
Do not assume they are normal.
Do not wait for them to worsen.

Early action makes a real difference.

Chapter Summary

COPD symptoms develop gradually and are often overlooked

Shortness of breath is the most common symptom

Chronic cough and sputum production are important signs

Fatigue is a common but underrecognized symptom

Wheezing and chest tightness may occur

Frequent infections can indicate underlying lung disease

Patients often adapt their lifestyle without realizing it

Early recognition leads to better outcomes

Action Plan for You

Pay attention to your symptoms
Notice even mild changes

Do not ignore persistent cough or breathlessness
These are not normal

Seek early medical evaluation
Early diagnosis improves outcomes

Stay aware of changes in activity level
Reduced stamina is an important signal

Take symptoms seriously
Your body is trying to tell you something

Transition to Next Chapter

Now that you can recognize the symptoms of COPD, the next step is understanding how doctors make the diagnosis. In the next chapter, we will go deeper into the evaluation process and how COPD is confirmed.

CHAPTER 4: How COPD Is Diagnosed – Getting Clarity Early

Why Diagnosis Matters More Than You Think

In my practice, I have seen two common problems.

Some patients are told they have COPD without proper testing.
Others have COPD for years but are never diagnosed.

Both situations create confusion and delay proper care.

A clear diagnosis is not just a label. It is the foundation of everything that follows.

When the diagnosis is correct:

Treatment becomes focused

Progression can be slowed

Patients feel more confident and informed

Without clarity, everything else becomes uncertain.

It Starts with a Simple Conversation

Diagnosis does not begin with machines. It begins with listening.

When I see a patient, I start with a detailed history.

I ask about:

Breathlessness and how it has changed over time

Cough and sputum

Smoking history

Exposure to dust, fumes, or pollution

Past respiratory illnesses

Often, patients reveal important clues without realizing it.

For example:
"I avoid stairs now."
"I walk slower than before."

These small details help build the picture.

The Physical Examination – Useful but Limited

A physical examination is the next step.

Doctors may listen for:

Wheezing

Reduced breath sounds

Signs of air trapping

But here is something important.

In early COPD, the physical exam may be completely normal.

That is why we do not rely on examination alone.

Spirometry – The Most Important Test

If there is one test that defines COPD, it is spirometry.

This is a simple, quick breathing test that provides essential information.

During the test:

You take a deep breath

Then blow out as hard and fast as possible into a device

The machine measures how much air you can exhale and how quickly.

It may feel slightly uncomfortable for a few seconds, but it is safe and very informative.

Understanding the Key Measurements

Spirometry gives us important numbers.

The two most important are:

FEV1: The amount of air you can blow out in the first second

FVC: The total amount of air you can blow out

We also look at the ratio between these two.

In COPD:

The airways are narrowed

Airflow is limited

So the amount of air exhaled quickly is reduced

If the ratio remains low even after medication, it confirms airflow obstruction.

You do not need to remember the numbers.

What matters is this.

Spirometry gives objective proof of the condition.

Why Testing Is Done Before and After Medication

Spirometry is often repeated after giving a bronchodilator.

This helps answer an important question:

Can the airflow improve significantly?

In asthma, airflow often improves noticeably

In COPD, the improvement is usually limited

This helps distinguish between the two conditions.

Why COPD Is Sometimes Misdiagnosed

Despite available tests, errors still occur.

Common mistakes include:

Diagnosing COPD without spirometry

Assuming all smokers with cough have COPD

Confusing COPD with asthma

Misreading test results

These errors can lead to wrong treatment.

That is why proper testing is essential.

Why COPD Is Often Missed

Just as COPD can be overdiagnosed, it is also frequently missed.

Many patients:

Ignore early symptoms

Adjust their lifestyle without realizing it

Do not seek medical care

Even when they do, spirometry may not always be performed.

As a result, diagnosis is delayed.

Looking at the Whole Picture

A proper diagnosis is not based on one test alone.

It includes:

Symptoms

Risk factors

Spirometry results

Overall health

Each part adds to the overall understanding.

This approach ensures accuracy.

Additional Tests – When They Are Needed

Once COPD is suspected or confirmed, additional tests may be done.

These include:

Chest X-ray

CT scan

Oxygen level measurement

Blood tests

These tests help:

Rule out other conditions

Assess severity

Identify complications

But they do not replace spirometry.

A Practical Example

I recall a patient who had been treated for asthma for several years.

His symptoms were not improving as expected.

We performed spirometry, and the results clearly showed COPD.

After adjusting his treatment:

His symptoms improved

His flare-ups reduced

The correct diagnosis made all the difference.

Why Early Diagnosis Changes Outcomes

When COPD is diagnosed early:

Smoking cessation becomes more effective

Treatment begins sooner

Lung function decline slows

Quality of life is preserved

Delayed diagnosis reduces these benefits.

What This Means for You

If you have symptoms or risk factors, do not rely on assumptions.

Ask for proper evaluation.

Spirometry is simple, widely available, and extremely valuable.

Clarity at this stage changes everything that follows.

How COPD Is Diagnosed

Doctors use various tests to diagnose COPD. Here are the key steps involved in identifying the condition:

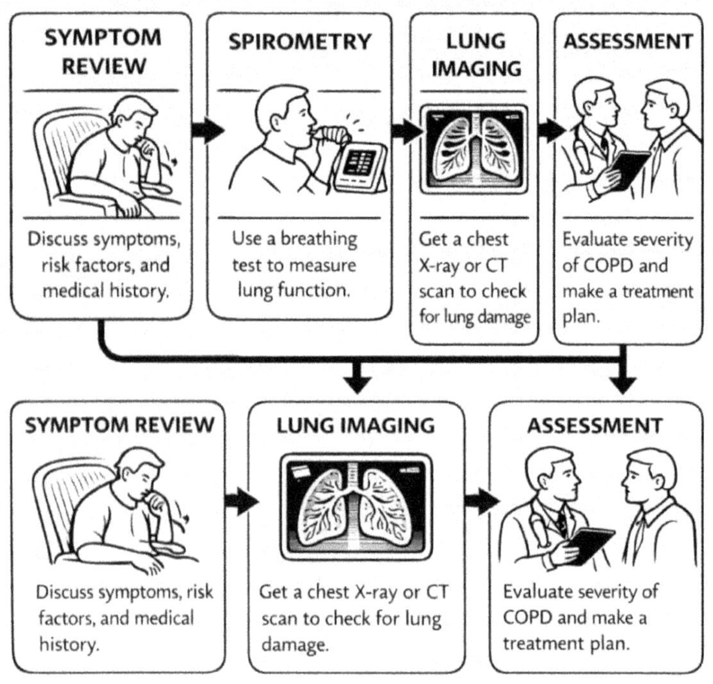

Chapter Summary

Accurate diagnosis is essential for effective treatment

History and symptom evaluation provide important clues

Physical examination alone is not enough

Spirometry is the key test for COPD

FEV1 and FVC help identify airflow limitation

Testing before and after medication distinguishes COPD from asthma

COPD is often misdiagnosed or missed

Additional tests help assess severity and complications

Early diagnosis improves long-term outcomes

Action Plan for You

Do not rely on assumptions
Symptoms alone cannot confirm COPD

Ask for spirometry if needed
It is the most important test

Understand your diagnosis
Ask your doctor to explain results clearly

Follow through with recommended tests
They provide valuable information

Act early
Early diagnosis leads to better outcomes

Transition to Next Chapter

Now that you understand how COPD is diagnosed, the next important step is knowing when it may not be COPD. In the next chapter, we will discuss other conditions that can mimic COPD and why correct diagnosis is so important.

CHAPTER 5: When It Is Not COPD – Conditions That Can Look Similar

Why This Chapter Is So Important

Not every patient with breathlessness has COPD.

This may sound obvious, but in real practice, this is where mistakes often happen.

I have seen patients treated for COPD for years when the real problem was something else. I have also seen patients with COPD being treated for the wrong condition.

Both situations delay proper care.

That is why this chapter is important.

Understanding what COPD is not can be just as valuable as understanding what it is.

Why So Many Conditions Look Alike

Many diseases affect breathing.

They can cause:

Shortness of breath

Cough

Fatigue

These symptoms overlap.

Without proper evaluation, it is easy to confuse one condition with another.

This is why diagnosis must always be careful and systematic.

Asthma – The Most Common Confusion

Asthma and COPD are often confused.

They share several symptoms:

Breathlessness

Wheezing

Cough

But there are important differences.

Asthma usually:

Starts earlier in life

Varies from day to day

Improves significantly with treatment

COPD usually:

Develops later in life

Progresses gradually

Does not fully reverse with treatment

Some patients have features of both. This is called overlap and needs special attention.

Heart Disease – A Frequently Missed Cause

The heart and lungs work closely together.

When the heart is not functioning properly, patients may feel breathless.

Conditions such as heart failure can cause:

Shortness of breath

Fatigue

Reduced exercise tolerance

Clues that suggest a heart problem include:

Swelling in the legs

Difficulty breathing when lying flat

Sudden weight gain due to fluid

Treating the heart condition can significantly improve symptoms.

Bronchiectasis – Chronic Cough with Mucus

Bronchiectasis is another lung condition that can resemble COPD.

It is characterized by:

Damaged and widened airways

Persistent cough

Large amounts of mucus

Frequent infections

Compared to COPD, sputum production is often more prominent.

CT scans help confirm the diagnosis.

Interstitial Lung Disease – A Different Pattern

In this group of diseases, the problem lies in the lung tissue, not the airways.

Patients often experience:

Breathlessness

Dry cough

Reduced ability to expand the lungs

Unlike COPD:

The lungs become stiff

Airflow is not the main issue

Treatment is completely different, which makes correct diagnosis essential.

Obesity and Deconditioning – A Common Situation

Not all breathlessness is due to disease.

In some patients:

Excess weight increases the effort of breathing

Lack of physical activity reduces stamina

This combination leads to significant breathlessness.

The important point is this.

Lung tests may be normal in these patients.

The focus should be on weight management and increasing activity.

Vocal Cord Dysfunction – Often Misunderstood

In this condition, the vocal cords do not open properly during breathing.

This can cause:

Sudden breathlessness

Noisy breathing

A sensation of choking

It is often mistaken for asthma or COPD.

Specialized evaluation is required for diagnosis.

Conditions That Can Mimic COPD

Other conditions can cause symptoms similar to COPD. It's important to distinguish between them to get the right teatment.

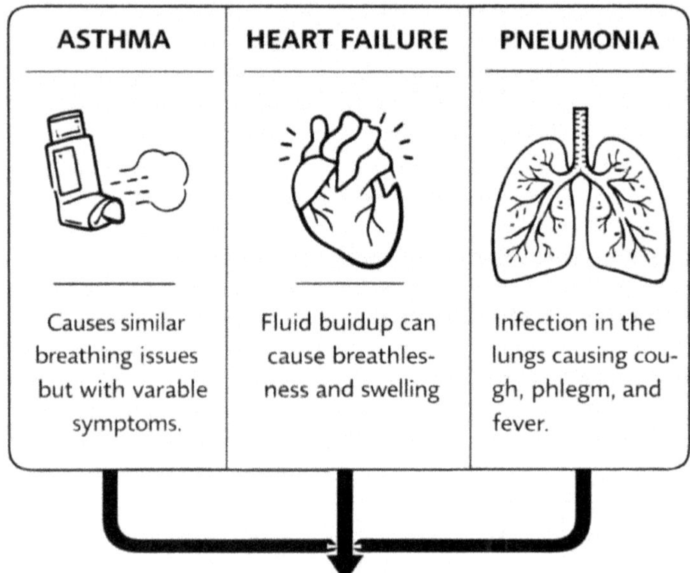

Lung Cancer – A Serious Condition to Consider

Some symptoms of lung cancer overlap with COPD.

These include:

Persistent cough

Weight loss

Breathlessness

In patients with risk factors, especially smokers, this possibility must always be considered.

Early detection is critical.

Pulmonary Embolism – A Sudden Emergency

A pulmonary embolism is a blood clot in the lungs.

It usually presents with:

Sudden breathlessness

Chest pain

Rapid heart rate

This is very different from COPD, which develops gradually.

This condition requires urgent medical attention.

Gastroesophageal Reflux and Chronic Cough

Acid reflux can sometimes cause:

Chronic cough

Throat irritation

A feeling of breathlessness

Patients may not realize the connection.

Treating reflux can improve symptoms.

When More Than One Condition Exists

In real life, patients often have more than one condition.

For example:

COPD with heart disease

COPD with asthma

COPD with obesity

This overlap can make symptoms more complex.

Treatment must address all contributing factors.

A Practical Example

I once treated a patient who had been labeled as having COPD for years.

Despite treatment, his symptoms continued to worsen.

On further evaluation, we found that heart failure was the main issue.

After proper treatment:

His breathing improved significantly

His energy levels increased

This case highlights an important lesson.

Correct diagnosis changes everything.

How Doctors Reach the Right Diagnosis

A proper diagnosis involves:

Careful history

Physical examination

Spirometry

Imaging when needed

Additional tests if required

Each step adds clarity.

Rushing the process increases the risk of error.

Why This Matters for You

As a patient, you should not try to diagnose yourself.

But you should stay aware.

If:

Symptoms do not improve

Treatment does not seem effective

it is reasonable to ask questions.

Sometimes, a second look reveals a different answer.

Chapter Summary

Many conditions can mimic COPD

Asthma is the most commonly confused condition

Heart disease is an important alternative cause

Other lung diseases such as bronchiectasis and interstitial lung disease may resemble COPD

Obesity and inactivity can cause breathlessness

Serious conditions like lung cancer and pulmonary embolism must be considered

Some patients have more than one condition

Accurate diagnosis requires careful evaluation

Action Plan for You

Do not assume all breathlessness is COPD
Be open to proper evaluation

Share complete information with your doctor
Details matter

Ask questions if treatment is not helping
This may indicate another condition

Stay alert to warning signs
Sudden symptoms need urgent attention

Follow through with recommended tests
They ensure accurate diagnosis

Transition to Next Chapter

Now that you understand what COPD is and what it is not, the next step is to understand how severe it is in your case. In the next chapter, we will discuss how COPD is classified and how doctors assess risk and progression.

CHAPTER 6: Understanding Severity and Risk – Where Do You Stand?

Why Knowing Your Stage Matters

Once COPD is diagnosed, most patients feel a sense of relief.

Finally, there is an answer.

But the next question naturally follows:

"How serious is it?"

This is an important question. Because COPD is not the same in every patient.

Some people have mild symptoms and live comfortably for years. Others experience frequent flare-ups and greater limitations.

Understanding where you stand helps guide:

Treatment decisions

Lifestyle changes

Long-term planning

It brings clarity to your condition.

COPD Is Not Defined by One Number

In the past, COPD severity was judged mainly by lung function numbers.

Today, we know that this approach is incomplete.

Two patients may have similar test results but very different symptoms.

For example:

One patient may walk comfortably

Another may struggle with daily activities

This is why modern assessment looks at the whole picture.

The Four Key Areas Doctors Evaluate

To understand severity, we look at four important factors:

Symptoms

Flare-up history

Lung function

Overall health

Each of these provides a piece of the puzzle.

Symptoms – What You Feel Every Day

Your daily symptoms are very important.

Doctors often use simple tools to measure them.

Breathlessness Scale (mMRC)

This focuses on how easily you become short of breath.

For example:

Do you feel breathless only with heavy activity

Or even while walking on level ground

COPD Assessment Test (CAT)

This looks at a broader range of symptoms, including:

Cough

Sputum

Chest tightness

Energy levels

Sleep

These tools help translate your experience into something measurable.

Flare-Ups – A Key Indicator of Risk

One of the strongest predictors of future problems is your history of flare-ups.

If you have:

Frequent exacerbations

Severe episodes requiring hospitalization

your risk of future complications is higher.

Each flare-up can:

Reduce lung function

Increase inflammation

Affect overall health

This is why preventing flare-ups is a major goal of treatment.

Lung Function – Still Important

Lung function testing, especially FEV1, remains important.

It helps us understand:

The degree of airflow limitation

The stage of the disease

However, it is only one part of the assessment.

It should not be used alone.

GOLD Classification – A Practical System

To simplify decision-making, patients are grouped using the GOLD system.

This system considers:

Symptom severity

Flare-up risk

Patients are placed into categories that help guide treatment.

In simple terms:

Some patients have mild symptoms and low risk

Others have more symptoms or frequent flare-ups

This classification helps doctors choose the most appropriate treatment.

The Role of Blood Tests

In some cases, blood tests provide additional guidance.

One important marker is the **eosinophil count**.

This helps:

Predict response to certain medications

Guide the use of inhaled steroids

This is part of a more personalized approach to treatment.

Looking Beyond the Lungs

COPD affects more than just breathing.

Many patients also have:

Heart disease

Diabetes

Anxiety or depression

Muscle weakness

These conditions influence how COPD behaves.

That is why assessment must include the whole person, not just the lungs.

Functional Ability – What You Can Actually Do

Numbers are important, but real-life function matters more.

Ask yourself:

How far can I walk

Can I perform daily tasks easily

Am I becoming less active

These practical aspects often reflect severity better than test results alone.

A Practical Example

Let me give you a simple example.

Two patients have similar lung function results.

The first patient:

Has minimal symptoms

Rarely has flare-ups

Remains active

The second patient:

Feels breathless daily

Has frequent flare-ups

Avoids activity

Clearly, these patients require different approaches.

This is why severity is not defined by numbers alone.

Why This Assessment Matters for Treatment

Understanding severity helps answer important questions:

Who needs more intensive treatment

Who needs additional medications

Who requires closer follow-up

It allows treatment to be tailored to your specific needs.

What This Means for You

You should not focus only on test results.

Instead, understand your condition as a whole.

Ask your doctor:

How severe is my COPD

What is my risk of flare-ups

What can I do to stay stable

This knowledge helps you stay proactive.

Chapter Summary

COPD severity is not defined by a single number

Assessment includes symptoms, flare-ups, lung function, and overall health

Symptom scores help measure daily impact

Flare-up history is a key predictor of future risk

GOLD classification helps guide treatment

Lung function remains important but is not the only factor

Blood tests may help personalize treatment

Functional ability reflects real-life severity

Action Plan for You

Understand your symptom level
Notice how COPD affects your daily life

Track flare-ups
Frequency and severity matter

Ask about your classification
It helps guide treatment

Stay engaged in your care
Your input is essential

Focus on overall health
Managing other conditions improves outcomes

Transition to Next Chapter

Now that you understand how COPD severity is assessed, the next important step is to understand the tests that help guide this evaluation. In the next chapter, we will look at the key investigations used in COPD and what they really mean for you.

CHAPTER 7: Important Tests That Guide Your Care – What They Mean for You

Why More Tests Are Needed After Diagnosis

Once COPD is diagnosed, many patients ask me a very reasonable question:

“Doctor, if we already know I have COPD, why do I need more tests?”

It is a fair question.

Spirometry confirms the diagnosis. But it does not tell us everything.

Additional tests help us:

Understand how advanced the disease is

Identify complications

Rule out other conditions

Plan treatment more precisely

Think of spirometry as the starting point. These tests help complete the picture.

Chest X-Ray – A Basic First Look

A chest X-ray is often one of the first tests performed.

It helps:

Rule out infections such as pneumonia

Detect lung masses or other abnormalities

Identify heart enlargement

Show signs of advanced lung changes

However, it is important to understand its limitation.

A chest X-ray can be normal in early COPD.

So it is helpful, but it cannot confirm the diagnosis by itself.

CT Scan – A Detailed View of the Lungs

A CT scan provides a much clearer and more detailed picture.

It can:

Detect emphysema

Show the distribution of lung damage

Identify bronchiectasis

Reveal conditions that may mimic COPD

In selected patients, a CT scan adds valuable information that cannot be seen on a standard X-ray.

But it is not required for every patient.

Lung Volume Testing – Measuring Trapped Air

Spirometry measures airflow, but it does not tell us how much air remains trapped in the lungs.

Lung volume tests help measure:

Total lung capacity

Residual air after exhalation

Degree of air trapping

This is important because air trapping is a key feature of COPD.

It explains why patients feel that they cannot fully empty their lungs.

Diffusion Capacity – How Well Oxygen Moves

Another important test measures how effectively oxygen moves from the lungs into the bloodstream.

This is called diffusion capacity.

In emphysema:

The air sacs are damaged

The surface area for gas exchange is reduced

As a result:

Oxygen transfer becomes less efficient

This test helps us understand the severity of this problem.

Measuring Oxygen Levels – A Critical Step

Oxygen levels are a vital part of COPD assessment.

There are two main ways to measure them.

Pulse Oximetry

A small device placed on your finger

Quick and painless

Gives an estimate of oxygen levels

Arterial Blood Gas (ABG)

A blood test taken from an artery

More precise measurement

Shows oxygen, carbon dioxide, and blood acidity

ABG is usually done in more advanced cases or during flare-ups.

Understanding COPD Tests

Doctors use several tests to evaluate COPD and determine its severity. Here's what each test measures and its significance:

SPIROMETRY	PULSE OXIMETRY	CHEST X-RAY / CT SCAN	BLOOD TESTS
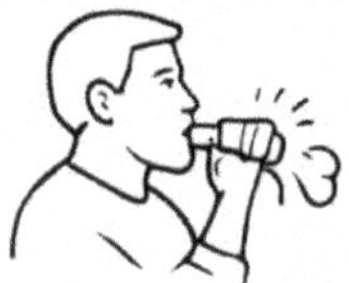	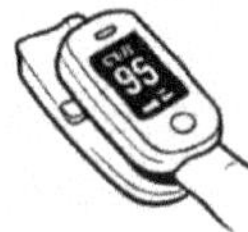	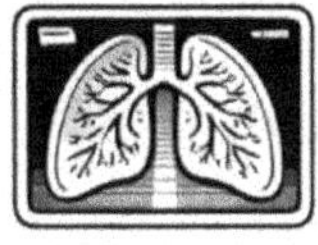	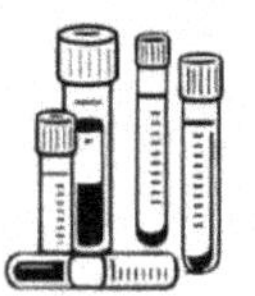
Measures how well your lungs work by checking airflow. Low FEV_1 indicates obstructed airflow and reduced lung function.	Checks oxygen saturation lev-els. Low SpO_2 (below 90%) indicates low oxygen in the blood.	Looks for lung damage, such as hyperinflation, air trapping, or other lung problems.	Identifies infect–ions, high carbon dioxide levels (hypercapnia), or other issues indicating COPD complications.

Exercise Testing – What Happens When You Move

Some patients feel fine at rest but become breathless with activity.

Exercise testing helps us understand:

How your body responds to activity

Whether oxygen levels drop during exertion

Your overall functional capacity

A simple example is the **six-minute walk test**.

It measures how far you can walk and how your oxygen levels behave during activity.

This provides very practical information.

Sleep Evaluation – When Breathing Changes at Night

Some patients experience breathing problems during sleep.

This may include:

Low oxygen levels at night

Interrupted sleep

Overlap with sleep apnea

In such cases, a sleep study may be recommended.

Improving sleep can significantly improve daytime energy and overall well-being.

Blood Tests – Looking for Additional Clues

Blood tests are often used to support evaluation.

They may include:

Eosinophil count to guide treatment

Hemoglobin levels

Markers of infection

In selected patients, testing for **alpha-1 antitrypsin deficiency** may be done.

These tests help personalize treatment.

Screening for Complications

COPD can affect other parts of the body.

Doctors may evaluate for:

Heart disease

Pulmonary hypertension

Osteoporosis

Muscle weakness

Identifying these conditions early improves overall care.

Not Every Patient Needs Every Test

It is important to understand that not all tests are required for every patient.

The choice depends on:

Severity of symptoms

Stage of disease

Presence of complications

Treatment planning

A mild case may require only basic testing. More advanced cases may need detailed evaluation.

A Practical Example

I recall a patient who had moderate COPD based on spirometry.

However, his symptoms were more severe than expected.

We performed additional tests, including a CT scan and diffusion study.

These showed significant emphysema and reduced oxygen transfer.

This helped us adjust his treatment and monitor him more closely.

Without these tests, we might have underestimated his condition.

Why These Tests Matter to You

These tests are not done just to generate reports.

They answer important questions:

How severe is the disease

What type of COPD is present

Are there complications

What treatment is most appropriate

When used properly, they provide clarity and direction.

What You Should Remember

You do not need to remember every test.

What matters is understanding their purpose.

Each test adds a piece to the overall picture of your health.

Chapter Summary

Spirometry confirms COPD but does not provide complete information

Chest X-ray helps rule out other conditions

CT scan provides detailed imaging of lung damage

Lung volume tests measure air trapping

Diffusion capacity assesses oxygen transfer

Oxygen levels are measured with pulse oximetry or ABG

Exercise testing evaluates functional capacity

Sleep studies may be needed in selected patients

Blood tests help guide treatment decisions

Testing is tailored to individual needs

Action Plan for You

Understand why tests are recommended
Each test has a purpose

Do not hesitate to ask questions
Clarity reduces anxiety

Follow through with testing
It improves diagnosis and treatment

Keep records of your results
Helps track progress over time

Focus on the bigger picture
Tests are tools to improve your care

Transition to Next Chapter

Now that you understand the tests used in COPD, the next important step is learning about flare-ups. In the next chapter, we will discuss what flare-ups are, why they happen, and how to recognize and manage them early.

CHAPTER 8: Flare-Ups in COPD – Recognizing and Acting Early

Why Flare-Ups Deserve Special Attention

If there is one aspect of COPD that can quickly change the course of the disease, it is a flare-up.

Many patients use different words:

"My breathing suddenly got worse"

"I had an attack"

"I could not catch my breath"

In medical terms, we call this an **exacerbation** or flare-up.

These episodes are not minor events.

Each flare-up can:

Worsen symptoms

Reduce lung function

Increase the risk of hospitalization

Affect long-term health

This is why recognizing and managing flare-ups early is so important.

What Exactly Is a Flare-Up

A flare-up is a sudden worsening of your usual COPD symptoms.

It goes beyond your normal day-to-day variation.

Common features include:

Increased breathlessness

More frequent or severe coughing

Change in sputum amount or color

Chest tightness

Fatigue

These changes may develop over hours or a few days.

The key is this.

You know your normal. A flare-up is when things clearly move away from that baseline.

Why Flare-Ups Happen

There are several common triggers.

Infections

This is the most frequent cause.

Viral infections such as colds

Bacterial infections

These lead to increased inflammation in the airways.

Air Pollution

Exposure to polluted air can irritate the lungs and trigger symptoms.

Weather Changes

Cold air or sudden temperature changes may worsen breathing in some patients.

Missed Medications

Skipping regular inhalers can reduce control and increase the risk of flare-ups.

Other Medical Conditions

Heart problems or other illnesses can sometimes mimic or trigger worsening symptoms.

Early Warning Signs – The Most Important Tool

One of the most powerful things you can learn is to recognize early warning signs.

These include:

Slight increase in breathlessness

Needing your rescue inhaler more often

Change in sputum color

Feeling more tired than usual

These changes may seem small, but they are often the beginning of a flare-up.

Acting at this stage can prevent the situation from worsening.

How Flare-Ups Progress If Ignored

If early signs are not addressed, symptoms may worsen.

Breathing becomes more difficult

Activity becomes limited

Anxiety increases

Oxygen levels may drop

In severe cases:

Hospitalization may be required

This progression is often preventable with early action.

What You Should Do at the First Sign

Every patient should have a clear action plan.

At the first sign of worsening:

Use your rescue inhaler as instructed

Increase medications if advised by your doctor

Rest and avoid overexertion

Monitor your symptoms closely

These steps may seem simple, but they are very effective.

When to Contact Your Doctor

Do not wait too long.

You should contact your doctor if:

Symptoms do not improve within 24–48 hours

Breathlessness continues to worsen

Sputum becomes thick, yellow, or green

You develop fever

Early medical treatment can prevent complications.

When It Is an Emergency

Some situations require immediate medical attention.

Seek urgent care if:

You are extremely breathless

You cannot speak full sentences

You feel confused or drowsy

Your lips or fingertips appear bluish

Do not delay in these situations.

Treatment of Flare-Ups

Depending on severity, treatment may include:

Short-acting bronchodilators

Oral steroids

Antibiotics if infection is suspected

Oxygen therapy

In severe cases, hospital care may be required.

The earlier treatment begins, the better the outcome.

Preventing Future Flare-Ups

Prevention is always better than treatment.

Key strategies include:

Taking medications regularly

Staying up to date with vaccinations

Avoiding exposure to pollutants

Practicing good hand hygiene

Maintaining physical activity

Patients who follow these steps often experience fewer flare-ups.

Recognizing a COPD Flare-Up

A COPD flare-up, or exacerbation, is when symptoms worsen suddenly. Recognizing early warning signs and knowing when to act can prevent serious complications:

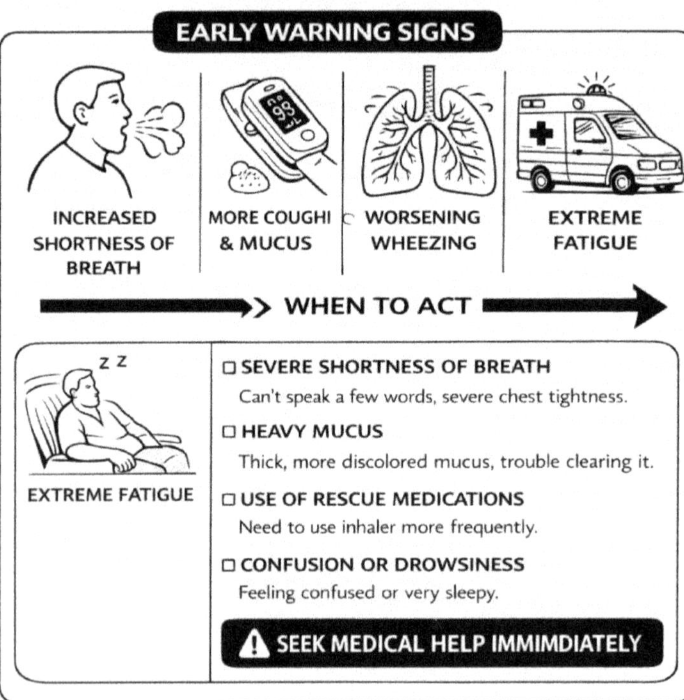

The Emotional Impact of Flare-Ups

Flare-ups are not just physical events.

They can be frightening.

Patients may feel:

Anxiety

Loss of control

Fear of recurrence

Understanding what is happening and having a plan reduces this fear.

A Practical Example

I remember a patient who used to wait until symptoms became severe before seeking help.

He had frequent hospitalizations.

We worked on recognizing early signs and acting quickly.

Over time:

His flare-ups became less severe

Hospital visits reduced

His confidence improved

The disease did not disappear, but his control over it improved significantly.

Why Early Action Changes Everything

The difference between a mild flare-up and a severe one often comes down to timing.

Early action:

Reduces severity

Shortens recovery time

Prevents complications

Delaying action allows the problem to grow.

What This Means for You

You are the first person to notice changes in your body.

Do not ignore them.

Do not wait for symptoms to become severe.

Your awareness and timely action are your strongest tools.

Chapter Summary

Flare-ups are sudden worsening of COPD symptoms

They are serious and can affect long-term health

Common triggers include infections, pollution, and missed medications

Early warning signs are often subtle but important

Acting early can prevent severe episodes

Clear action plans improve outcomes

Some symptoms require urgent medical attention

Prevention strategies reduce frequency of flare-ups

Action Plan for You

Learn your early warning signs
Small changes matter

Use your action plan
Act quickly when symptoms worsen

Do not delay medical care
Early treatment is more effective

Stay consistent with medications
Prevention is key

Reduce exposure to triggers
Protect your lungs daily

Transition to Next Chapter

Now that you understand flare-ups and how to manage them, the next important step is treatment. In the next chapter, we will begin discussing medications used in COPD, starting with inhalers, which form the foundation of treatment.

CHAPTER 9: Medications in COPD – Understanding the Foundation of Treatment

Why Medications Matter

Once COPD is diagnosed, one of the first things patients ask is:

“Doctor, what medicines will I need?”

This is an important question, but it is equally important to understand something else.

Medications do not cure COPD.

What they do is:

Open the airways

Reduce symptoms

Prevent flare-ups

Improve quality of life

When used correctly, they can make a meaningful difference in how you feel and function every day.

Two Main Goals of Treatment

COPD medications are designed with two clear goals in mind:

Relieve symptoms

Prevent worsening of the disease

Some medicines work quickly to relieve breathlessness. Others work slowly but help keep the disease under control.

Both are important.

Understanding the Two Types of Inhalers

Most COPD medications are given through inhalers.

These are broadly divided into two types:

Rescue Inhalers (Quick Relief)

These are used when you suddenly feel breathless.

They:

Work quickly

Relax the airway muscles

Provide rapid relief

Patients often carry them for immediate use.

Understanding a COPD Medications

Medications are used to help manage symptoms, prevent flare-ups, and improve the quality of life in COPD. Here's a look at the main types:

EARLY WARNING SIGNS

BRONCHODILATORS

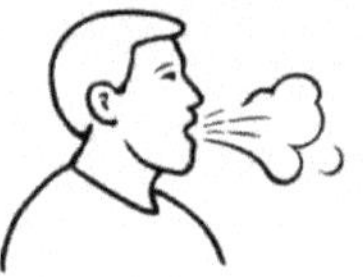

- Relax and open the airways
- Short-or long-acting types

INHALED CORTICOSTEROIDS

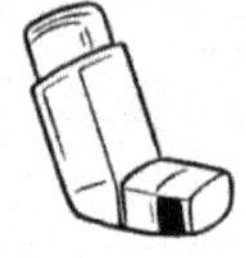

- Reduce airway inflammation
- For frequent flare-ups

COMBINATION INHALERS

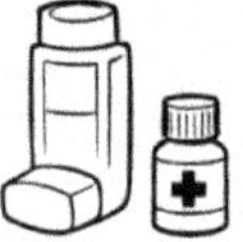

- Contain bronchod-dilators and steroids
- Convenient combined treatment

OTHER MEDICATIONS

- ☐ **Oral Steroids:** Used short-term for severe flare-ups
- ☐ **Mucolytics:** Help thin and loosen mucus
- ☐ **Antibiotics:** Treat bacterial infections

Maintenance Inhalers (Daily Use)

These are taken regularly, even when you feel well.

They:

Keep the airways open

Reduce inflammation

Prevent symptoms and flare-ups

Many patients make the mistake of using them only when needed.

That reduces their effectiveness.

Bronchodilators – Opening the Airways

The most important group of medications in COPD is bronchodilators.

They work by relaxing the muscles around the airways.

This leads to:

Wider airways

Easier airflow

Reduced breathlessness

There are two main types:

Short-Acting Bronchodilators

Provide quick relief

Used as needed

Act within minutes

These are your "rescue" medications.

Long-Acting Bronchodilators

Work for many hours

Taken regularly

Help maintain stable breathing

These are the backbone of daily treatment.

Inhaled Steroids – Reducing Inflammation

In some patients, inflammation plays a significant role.

Inhaled steroids help by:

Reducing airway inflammation

Decreasing flare-ups

They are not required for every patient.

They are usually recommended for:

Patients with frequent flare-ups

Patients with certain blood test findings

Using them unnecessarily may increase side effects, so proper selection is important.

Combination Inhalers – Simplifying Treatment

Many patients use inhalers that combine different medications.

These may include:

Two bronchodilators

A bronchodilator plus a steroid

Combination inhalers:

Improve convenience

Increase effectiveness

Reduce the number of devices needed

They are commonly used in moderate to severe COPD.

Oral Medications – Used in Selected Cases

While inhalers are the mainstay, some patients may need oral medications.

These include:

Anti-inflammatory drugs

Medications to reduce flare-ups

They are usually added when inhalers alone are not enough.

Antibiotics – Only When Needed

Antibiotics are not used routinely.

They are prescribed when:

There is a bacterial infection

Sputum becomes yellow or green

Fever is present

Using antibiotics unnecessarily can cause harm, so they should be used carefully.

Steroid Tablets – For Flare-Ups

Oral steroids are often used during flare-ups.

They:

Reduce inflammation quickly

Improve symptoms

However, long-term use is avoided because of side effects.

Why Correct Inhaler Use Is Critical

This is one of the most important points in COPD care.

Even the best medication will not work if the inhaler is used incorrectly.

Common mistakes include:

Poor inhalation technique

Incorrect timing

Skipping doses

Studies show that many patients do not use inhalers properly.

This reduces the benefit of treatment.

Adherence – Taking Medicines Regularly

Another common issue is inconsistency.

Patients may:

Skip doses when they feel better

Use medications irregularly

This leads to:

Poor symptom control

Increased flare-ups

Consistency is essential.

Side Effects – What You Should Know

Most COPD medications are safe when used correctly.

However, some side effects may occur.

For example:

Tremor with bronchodilators

Dry mouth

Throat irritation with inhaled steroids

These are usually mild and manageable.

Discuss any concerns with your doctor.

A Practical Example

I remember a patient who felt that his medications were not helping.

On reviewing his inhaler technique, we found that he was not inhaling properly.

After correcting the technique:

His symptoms improved significantly

His need for rescue inhaler reduced

The medication had not changed. The way it was used had changed.

Why Understanding Your Medications Matters

When you understand your treatment:

You use it correctly

You follow it consistently

You feel more confident

This leads to better outcomes.

What This Means for You

Do not think of medications as a burden.

Think of them as tools that help you:

Breathe better

Stay active

Prevent complications

Using them properly makes all the difference.

Chapter Summary

COPD medications relieve symptoms and prevent worsening

Inhalers are the main form of treatment

Rescue inhalers provide quick relief

Maintenance inhalers are used daily

Bronchodilators open the airways

Inhaled steroids reduce inflammation in selected patients

Combination inhalers improve convenience and effectiveness

Oral medications are used in specific situations

Correct inhaler technique is essential

Consistent use improves outcomes

Action Plan for You

Know your medications
Understand what each one does

Use inhalers correctly
Review your technique regularly

Take medications consistently
Do not skip doses

Use rescue inhaler when needed
Do not overuse

Discuss side effects with your doctor
Adjustments can be made

Transition to Next Chapter

Now that you understand the role of medications, the next important step is mastering how to use inhalers correctly. In the next chapter, we will go deeper into inhaler techniques and ensure you get the maximum benefit from your treatment.

CHAPTER 10: Inhalers Done Right – Getting the Full Benefit from Your Treatment

Why This Chapter Is More Important Than You Think

Let me be very direct.

Even the best COPD medication will not work if the inhaler is not used correctly.

This is one of the most common and most overlooked problems I see in practice.

Many patients believe they are taking their medications properly. But when I watch them use their inhaler, I often notice small mistakes.

These small mistakes lead to big problems:

Less medication reaches the lungs

Symptoms do not improve as expected

Patients feel frustrated

The solution is simple.

Learn the correct technique, and practice it consistently.

How Inhalers Actually Work

An inhaler is designed to deliver medication directly into the lungs.

This has several advantages:

Faster action

Lower doses compared to tablets

Fewer side effects

But for this to work, the medication must reach deep into the airways.

If the technique is incorrect:

Much of the medicine stays in the mouth or throat

Very little reaches the lungs

That is why technique matters so much.

The Basic Principles of Good Inhaler Use

No matter which inhaler you use, a few principles apply to all.

Start with a full exhalation

Inhale at the correct speed

Coordinate your breathing with the device

Hold your breath after inhalation

These steps ensure that the medicine reaches where it is needed.

Step-by-Step Technique (General Guide)

Although different inhalers have slightly different methods, this general approach works for most:

Sit or stand upright

Exhale fully

Place the inhaler properly in your mouth

Start inhaling slowly

Press the inhaler (if required)

Continue a slow, deep breath

Hold your breath for about 5–10 seconds

Exhale slowly

This entire process takes only a few seconds, but it makes a big difference.

Different Types of Inhalers

There are several types of inhalers.

Understanding your device helps you use it correctly.

Metered-Dose Inhalers (MDI)

These are the most common.

They release a fixed dose of medication when pressed.

Key challenge:

Coordinating pressing and inhaling at the same time

Dry Powder Inhalers (DPI)

These do not require pressing.

You inhale the medication as a powder.

Key point:

You need a strong, deep inhalation

Soft Mist Inhalers

These release a slow-moving mist.

They are easier to inhale and require less coordination.

Using a Spacer – Making It Easier

For patients using MDIs, a spacer can be very helpful.

A spacer is a simple attachment that:

Holds the medication

Allows you to inhale it more easily

Benefits include:

Better drug delivery

Less need for perfect timing

Reduced side effects

I often recommend spacers, especially for older patients.

Common Mistakes to Avoid

Let me highlight some of the most frequent errors:

Not exhaling before using the inhaler

Inhaling too fast or too slow

Poor coordination with MDIs

Not holding the breath long enough

Skipping doses

Not shaking the inhaler (for MDIs)

These mistakes are very common, but easily correctable.

Why Rinsing Your Mouth Matters

If you are using inhaled steroids, always rinse your mouth after use.

This helps:

Prevent throat irritation

Reduce the risk of fungal infections

It is a simple habit that makes a big difference.

Checking Your Technique Regularly

Even if you have been using an inhaler for years, it is a good idea to review your technique.

I often ask my patients:
"Show me how you use your inhaler."

This simple step helps identify and correct mistakes.

Adherence – Using It Every Day

Another issue is consistency.

Patients sometimes use inhalers only when they feel symptoms.

But maintenance inhalers are designed for daily use.

Skipping doses leads to:

Poor control

Increased flare-ups

Consistency is as important as technique.

A Practical Example

I remember a patient who said:

"Doctor, these inhalers are not helping me."

When I observed him, I noticed he was inhaling too quickly and not holding his breath.

We corrected his technique.

Within a few weeks:

His symptoms improved

He needed his rescue inhaler less often

The medicine had not changed.

The method had changed.

Why This Chapter Matters for You

If you take only one practical lesson from this book, let it be this.

Correct inhaler use is essential.

It is not complicated, but it requires attention and consistency.

What This Means for You

Take a few minutes to review your inhaler technique.

Ask your doctor or healthcare provider to watch you use it.

Small corrections can lead to significant improvement.

Chapter Summary

Inhaler technique is critical for effective treatment

Medication must reach the lungs to work properly

Basic steps include proper inhalation and breath holding

Different inhalers require slightly different techniques

Spacers can improve delivery for MDIs

Common mistakes are frequent but correctable

Rinsing the mouth after steroid inhalers is important

Regular review of technique improves outcomes

Consistent daily use is essential

Action Plan for You

Review your inhaler technique
Make sure you are using it correctly

Ask your doctor to check your technique
Small corrections matter

Use your inhalers consistently
Do not skip doses

Consider using a spacer if needed
It improves effectiveness

Rinse your mouth after steroid inhalers
Prevent side effects

Transition to Next Chapter

Now that you understand how to use inhalers correctly, the next step is to explore other important treatments beyond medications. In the next chapter, we will discuss non-drug treatments that play a powerful role in improving COPD symptoms and quality of life.

CHAPTER 11: Non-Drug Treatments – The Missing Piece in COPD Care

Why Medicines Alone Are Not Enough

Many patients believe that once they start inhalers, everything else will fall into place.

That is not how COPD works.

Medicines are important. They open the airways and reduce symptoms. But they do not build strength, improve stamina, or restore confidence.

That part depends on you.

In my experience, patients who combine medications with non-drug treatments do far better than those who rely on medicines alone.

This chapter focuses on those essential steps.

Pulmonary Rehabilitation – One of the Most Effective Treatments

If I had to choose one non-drug treatment that makes the biggest difference, it would be pulmonary rehabilitation.

This is a structured program that includes:

Supervised exercise

Breathing training

Education about COPD

Emotional support

Many patients hesitate at first.

They say:
"Doctor, I am already breathless. How can I exercise?"

But pulmonary rehabilitation is designed specifically for patients like you.

It starts gently and progresses gradually.

What Pulmonary Rehabilitation Achieves

Pulmonary rehabilitation does not cure COPD.

But it improves how your body functions with the condition.

Benefits include:

Better exercise tolerance

Reduced breathlessness

Increased muscle strength

Improved confidence

Many patients tell me:
"I feel stronger. I can do more than before."

That is a meaningful outcome.

Exercise – The Most Powerful Habit You Can Build

Exercise is not optional in COPD care.

It is essential.

When you avoid activity:

Muscles weaken

Endurance decreases

Breathlessness worsens

This creates a cycle.

You feel breathless, so you avoid activity. Then you become weaker, and breathlessness increases.

Exercise helps break this cycle.

Starting Exercise Safely

You do not need intense workouts.

Simple activities are enough.

Walking

Light strength training

Gentle stretching

The key is to start slowly.

For example:

Begin with 5–10 minutes of walking

Increase gradually over weeks

Consistency matters more than intensity.

Breathing Techniques – Simple but Effective

Certain breathing techniques can provide immediate relief.

Pursed-Lip Breathing

Inhale through your nose

Exhale slowly through pursed lips

This helps:

Keep airways open longer

Reduce air trapping

Improve breathing efficiency

Diaphragmatic Breathing

Focus on using your diaphragm rather than chest muscles

This makes breathing more efficient and less tiring.

Practicing these techniques regularly makes them easier to use during daily activities.

Energy Conservation – Doing More Without Exhaustion

COPD can make routine tasks tiring.

Learning to conserve energy is very helpful.

Practical strategies include:

Sitting while doing tasks

Breaking activities into smaller steps

Planning your day

Avoiding unnecessary movements

These small adjustments reduce strain and improve efficiency.

Nutrition – Supporting Your Body from Within

Breathing in COPD requires more energy.

This makes nutrition very important.

Some patients lose weight. Others gain weight due to reduced activity.

Both situations can worsen symptoms.

If You Are Underweight

Eat small, frequent meals

Focus on protein-rich foods

Include calorie-dense options

If You Are Overweight

Aim for gradual weight reduction

Combine diet with regular activity

Balanced nutrition supports strength and energy.

Vaccinations – Preventing Flare-Ups

Infections are a major cause of flare-ups.

Vaccinations reduce this risk.

Important vaccines include:

Influenza

Pneumococcal

COVID-19

RSV (in selected patients)

These vaccines do not eliminate risk completely, but they significantly reduce complications.

Self-Management – Taking an Active Role

COPD management does not happen only in the doctor's office.

It happens every day.

Self-management includes:

Taking medications regularly

Recognizing early symptoms

Following an action plan

Staying active

Patients who take an active role do better over time.

Emotional Health – An Important but Overlooked Area

Living with COPD can be stressful.

Patients may feel:

Anxiety

Fear of breathlessness

Frustration

These feelings are normal.

Support can come from:

Family

Support groups

Counseling

Addressing emotional health improves overall well-being.

A Practical Example

I remember a patient who depended entirely on medications.

He avoided activity because he feared breathlessness.

We introduced a simple plan:

Walking daily

Breathing exercises

Gradual increase in activity

Within months:

His stamina improved

His confidence returned

The medication did not change.

His approach changed.

Why These Treatments Are Often Overlooked

Despite their benefits, non-drug treatments are often underused.

Common reasons include:

Lack of awareness

Fear of exertion

Limited access to programs

But even simple steps at home can make a difference.

What This Means for You

Medicines help you breathe.

But these non-drug treatments help you live better.

They give you strength, confidence, and independence.

Chapter Summary

Non-drug treatments are essential in COPD care

Pulmonary rehabilitation improves function and confidence

Regular exercise breaks the cycle of inactivity

Breathing techniques reduce breathlessness

Energy conservation improves daily efficiency

Nutrition supports strength and health

Vaccinations reduce infection risk

Self-management improves long-term outcomes

Emotional health is an important part of care

Action Plan for You

Stay physically active
Start small and build gradually

Practice breathing techniques
Use them daily

Consider pulmonary rehabilitation
It can make a significant difference

Maintain proper nutrition
Support your body

Stay up to date with vaccinations
Prevent infections

Transition to Next Chapter

Now that you understand the importance of non-drug treatments, the next step is to learn about oxygen therapy and advanced support. In the next chapter, we will discuss when oxygen is needed and how it can improve your quality of life.

CHAPTER 12: Oxygen Therapy – When and How It Helps

Understanding the Need for Oxygen

One of the most emotional moments for many patients is when oxygen therapy is discussed.

I often hear:
"Doctor, does this mean my condition is very serious?"

Let me reassure you.

Oxygen is not a sign of failure. It is a form of support.

Just like glasses help you see better, oxygen helps your body function better when your lungs are not able to supply enough oxygen on their own.

The goal is simple.

To give your body what it needs.

Why Oxygen Is Essential for the Body

Every cell in your body depends on oxygen.

Your:

Brain

Heart

Muscles

all require a steady supply of oxygen to function properly.

When oxygen levels fall:

You feel tired

Your thinking may become less clear

Your heart has to work harder

Over time, low oxygen levels can strain multiple organs.

Providing supplemental oxygen helps prevent this.

When Is Oxygen Therapy Needed

Not every patient with COPD needs oxygen.

It is recommended only when oxygen levels in the blood are consistently low.

This is determined by:

Pulse oximetry

Arterial blood gas testing

Oxygen may be needed:

At rest

During activity

During sleep

The need varies from patient to patient.

Oxygen Therapy in COPD

Oxygen therapy is used for COPD patients with low blood oxygen levels. Here are the key facts about oxygen therapy and its benefits:

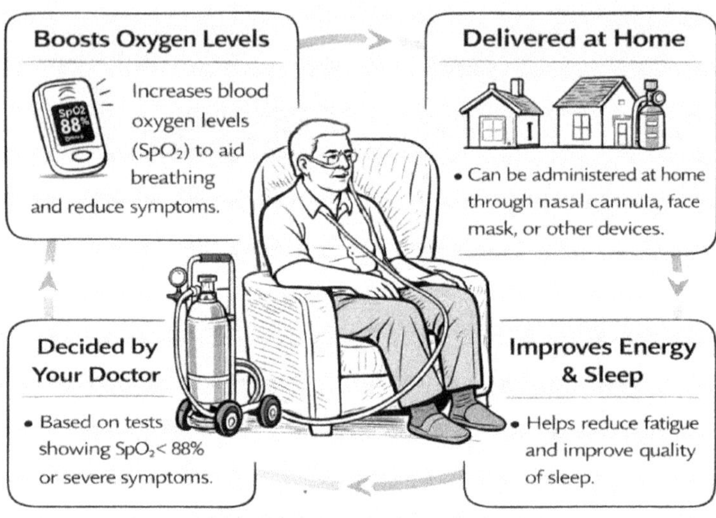

IMPORTANT:

1. **Avoid smoking** near oxygen.
2. Keep oxygen tanks upright and secure.
3. Follow your prescribed flow rate.

How Oxygen Therapy Helps

When used appropriately, oxygen therapy can:

Improve energy levels

Reduce breathlessness

Improve sleep quality

Protect the heart and other organs

Improve survival in selected patients

Many patients notice a clear improvement once oxygen is started.

Types of Oxygen Therapy

Oxygen therapy can be customized.

Continuous Oxygen

Used throughout the day and night for patients with persistently low oxygen levels.

Ambulatory Oxygen

Used during physical activity to maintain oxygen levels.

Nocturnal Oxygen

Used during sleep when oxygen levels drop at night.

The goal is to match oxygen use to your specific needs.

Common Concerns About Oxygen

Let us address a few common fears.

"Will I Become Dependent on Oxygen?"

No.

Oxygen is not addictive. It is prescribed because your body needs it.

"Will It Limit My Life?"

Not necessarily.

Modern portable systems allow many patients to:

Move around freely

Travel

Continue daily activities

"Does It Mean My Disease Is Very Advanced?"

Not always.

It simply means that your oxygen levels need support.

Living Safely with Oxygen

Safety is very important.

Key precautions include:

Never smoke near oxygen

Keep it away from open flames

Store equipment properly

Follow instructions carefully

Oxygen supports life, but it must be handled responsibly.

Different Oxygen Delivery Systems

There are different ways oxygen is delivered.

Oxygen Concentrators

Used at home

Extract oxygen from the air

Provide a continuous supply

Portable Oxygen Systems

Lightweight

Used for mobility and travel

Oxygen Cylinders

Store oxygen under pressure

Used as backup or for travel

Your doctor will help choose the most appropriate system.

Using Oxygen Correctly

To get the full benefit:

Use oxygen for the prescribed number of hours

Do not reduce use without advice

Ensure proper fit of nasal cannula or mask

Consistency is important.

Oxygen and Daily Life

Many patients initially feel self-conscious.

They worry about:

Appearance

Social situations

Dependence

But over time, most patients adapt.

They realize that oxygen allows them to:

Feel better

Do more

Stay active

Traveling with Oxygen

Travel is still possible.

With planning:

Portable devices can be used

Airlines can accommodate oxygen needs

Adequate supply can be arranged

Preparation is the key.

A Practical Example

I remember a patient who resisted oxygen therapy for months.

He felt it would restrict his life.

When he finally agreed:

His energy improved

He slept better

He became more active

He later said:
"I should have started earlier."

This is a very common experience.

Why Accepting Oxygen Matters

Delaying oxygen therapy when it is needed can lead to:

Increased strain on the heart

Worsening fatigue

Reduced quality of life

Accepting it at the right time improves outcomes.

What This Means for You

If oxygen is recommended:

Do not fear it.
Do not resist it unnecessarily.

Understand why it is needed and use it properly.

It is there to help you live better.

Chapter Summary

Oxygen therapy is used when blood oxygen levels are low

It supports vital organs and improves energy

Not all COPD patients require oxygen

Different types of oxygen therapy are available

Oxygen is not addictive

Modern systems allow mobility and independence

Safety precautions are essential

Proper and consistent use improves outcomes

Action Plan for You

Understand your oxygen levels
Know if and when you need oxygen

Use oxygen as prescribed
Consistency is important

Follow safety precautions
Protect yourself and others

Stay active
Oxygen should support your activity

Ask questions
Clarity reduces fear

Transition to Next Chapter

Now that you understand oxygen therapy, the next step is to explore advanced treatment options. In the next chapter, we will discuss procedures and surgical treatments, and when they may be considered in COPD.

CHAPTER 13: Procedures and Surgical Options – When Additional Help Is Needed

When Standard Treatment Is Not Enough

Most patients with COPD are managed effectively with:

Medications

Lifestyle changes

Pulmonary rehabilitation

But there are situations where, despite doing everything right, symptoms remain significant.

Patients may say:

"I cannot walk even short distances."

"Breathing feels like a constant struggle."

In such cases, we begin to consider additional options.

These include certain procedures and surgical treatments.

They are not needed for everyone. But for selected patients, they can make a meaningful difference.

Understanding the Goal of These Treatments

Before we discuss specific options, it is important to set the right expectations.

These procedures do not cure COPD.

Their purpose is to:

Improve breathing efficiency

Reduce symptoms

Enhance quality of life

In selected cases, they may also improve survival.

The key is proper patient selection.

Lung Volume Reduction Surgery – Creating Space to Breathe

In some patients with emphysema, parts of the lungs become severely damaged and overinflated.

These areas:

Do not function effectively

Trap air

Compress healthier lung tissue

Lung volume reduction surgery removes these damaged portions.

This allows:

Healthier lung areas to expand better

The diaphragm to function more efficiently

Breathing to become easier

Patients selected for this procedure undergo careful evaluation.

Endobronchial Valve Therapy – A Less Invasive Option

For patients who may not be candidates for surgery, a less invasive option is available.

Endobronchial valves are small devices placed inside the airways using a bronchoscope.

They work by:

Blocking airflow into the most damaged areas

Allowing trapped air to escape

This reduces hyperinflation and improves breathing.

Benefits may include:

Reduced breathlessness

Improved exercise capacity

Better quality of life

This procedure does not require open surgery.

Bullectomy – Removing Large Air Spaces

Some patients develop large air-filled spaces called bullae.

These:

Do not contribute to oxygen exchange

Compress surrounding lung tissue

In such cases, removing these bullae can:

Improve lung function

Reduce symptoms

This procedure is considered when the bullae are large and clearly affecting breathing.

Lung Transplant – A Major but Life-Changing Option

In advanced COPD, when other treatments are no longer effective, lung transplant may be considered.

This is a serious and complex decision.

A transplant involves:

Replacing diseased lungs with donor lungs

Lifelong follow-up

Use of medications to prevent rejection

For selected patients, it can:

Improve quality of life

Extend survival

However, it carries risks, including infection and rejection.

Who Is a Candidate for These Procedures

Not every patient is suitable for these treatments.

Selection depends on:

Type of COPD (especially emphysema)

Severity of symptoms

Overall health

Presence of other conditions

Detailed testing is required before making a decision.

Risks and Considerations

Every procedure carries some risk.

These may include:

Complications from surgery

Infection

Limited improvement in some cases

It is important to weigh:

Potential benefits

Possible risks

A clear discussion with your doctor is essential.

Procedures and Surgeries for COPD

In severe cases of COPD where medications are not enough, certain procedures may help. Here are the main procedures and surgeries used for COPD management:

LUNG VOLUME REDUCTION	ENDOBRONCHIAL VALVES	LUNG TRANSPLANT
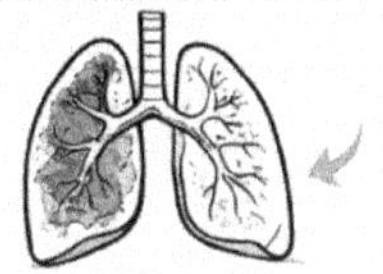 • Removes damaged lung tissue. • Improves breathing by reducing lung size.	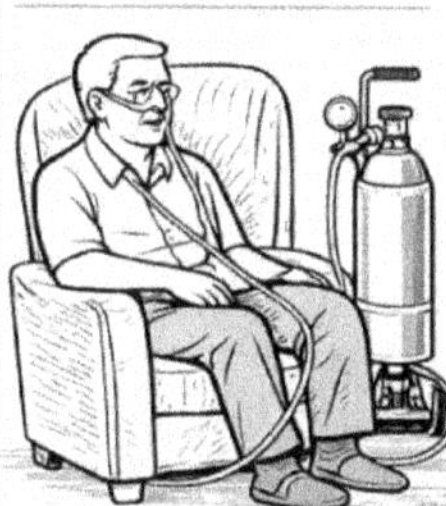	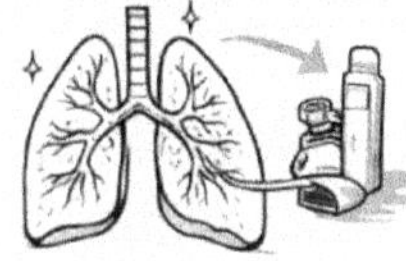 • Replaces diseased lungs with healthy donor lungs. • For end-stage COPD when other options fail.

CONSIDERATIONS:

- ✓ **Surgery** is considered when COPD is severe and other treatments don't work.
- ✓ **Doctors** evaluate risks and benefits based on the patient's health.
- ✓ **Requires** lifelong follow-up and medication.

Why These Options Are Not Commonly Used

You may wonder why these procedures are not offered to all patients.

The reasons include:

They are suitable only for selected patients

They require specialized centers

Benefits depend on proper selection

Most patients do well with standard treatment and do not need these interventions.

The Importance of Timing

Timing plays an important role.

Too early, and the risks may outweigh the benefits. Too late, and the patient may not be strong enough for the procedure.

Regular follow-up helps determine if and when such options should be considered.

A Practical Example

I remember a patient with severe emphysema who struggled despite optimal medical therapy.

After careful evaluation, he underwent a lung volume reduction procedure.

Over time:

His breathing improved

His activity level increased

His confidence returned

It was not a cure, but it was a meaningful improvement.

Why Awareness Matters

Even if you never need these procedures, it is important to know they exist.

They provide:

Additional options in advanced disease

Hope for selected patients

A more complete understanding of COPD care

What This Means for You

Focus first on:

Medications

Lifestyle changes

Rehabilitation

These help most patients.

But if symptoms remain severe, discuss advanced options with your doctor.

Chapter Summary

Most COPD patients are treated without surgery

Procedures are considered in selected cases

Lung volume reduction surgery removes damaged lung tissue

Endobronchial valves offer a less invasive option

Bullectomy helps in patients with large air spaces

Lung transplant is considered in advanced disease

Careful patient selection is essential

These treatments aim to improve quality of life

Action Plan for You

Focus on standard treatment first
Most patients do well without procedures

Attend regular follow-ups
This helps identify when additional options may be needed

Ask questions if symptoms remain severe
Explore all available options

Maintain overall health
This improves eligibility if procedures are needed

Stay informed
Knowledge helps you make better decisions

Transition to Next Chapter

Now that you understand advanced treatment options, the next important step is to look beyond the lungs. In the next chapter, we will discuss how COPD affects other parts of the body and why a whole-body approach is essential.

CHAPTER 14: COPD Beyond the Lungs – Why Whole-Body Care Matters

COPD Is Not Just a Lung Disease

When patients hear the word COPD, they naturally think about the lungs.

That is understandable.

But over the years, I have seen something very important.

COPD affects much more than breathing.

It influences the entire body.

If we focus only on the lungs and ignore the rest, we miss a large part of the problem.

And more importantly, we miss opportunities to improve health and quality of life.

Why COPD Affects the Whole Body

There are several reasons why COPD has widespread effects.

Chronic inflammation affects multiple systems

Reduced activity leads to muscle weakness

Low oxygen levels strain organs

COPD & Its Effects Beyond the Lungs

COPD not only affects the lungs, but can also have widespread effects on other organs in the body.

HEART

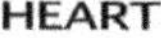

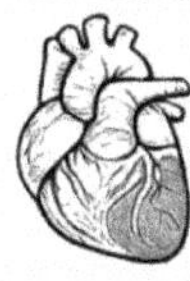

- Pulmonary hypertension
- Right heart strain (cor pulmonale)

BRAIN

- Low oxygen effects.
- Poor concentration
- Confusion in advanced disease.

MUSCLES

- Muscle weakness
- Reduced exercise tolerance
- Deconditioning.

BONES

- Osteoporosis risk
- Fracture risk.

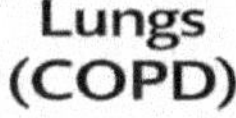

Lungs (COPD)

MOOD / MENTAL HEALTH

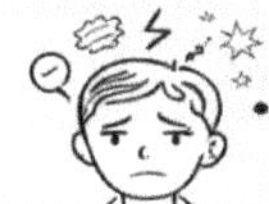

- Anxiety
- Depression

METABOLISM / WEIGHT

- Weight loss or muscle wasting in severe COPD.

MANAGING SYSTEMIC EFFECTS:

✓ Work closely with your healthcare provider.

✓ **Weight** loss or muscle wasting in severe COPD

Coexisting conditions are common

These factors work together.

The result is a condition that goes beyond the lungs.

Heart Health – A Close Connection

The heart and lungs are closely linked.

When the lungs are not working efficiently:

Oxygen levels may drop

The heart has to work harder

Over time, this can lead to:

Heart disease

Heart failure

Irregular heart rhythms

Many patients with COPD also have heart problems.

Sometimes, symptoms overlap, making diagnosis more complex.

Treating heart conditions properly can significantly improve overall symptoms.

Muscle Weakness – The Hidden Problem

One of the most overlooked effects of COPD is muscle weakness.

This happens because:

Physical activity decreases

The body uses more energy for breathing

Nutrition may be inadequate

Weak muscles make everyday activities more difficult.

Even simple tasks can feel exhausting.

This is why exercise and rehabilitation are so important.

Bone Health – The Risk of Osteoporosis

COPD increases the risk of osteoporosis.

Contributing factors include:

Reduced physical activity

Long-term use of certain medications

Nutritional deficiencies

Weak bones increase the risk of fractures.

A minor fall can lead to serious complications.

Maintaining bone health is an important part of care.

Weight Changes – Both Loss and Gain Matter

COPD affects body weight in different ways.

Some patients lose weight because:

Breathing requires extra energy

Appetite is reduced

Others gain weight due to inactivity.

Both situations can worsen symptoms.

Maintaining a healthy weight supports better breathing and overall health.

Anxiety and Depression – The Emotional Impact

Living with breathing difficulty can be stressful.

Patients often experience:

Anxiety during episodes of breathlessness

Fear of worsening symptoms

Frustration with limitations

Over time, this can lead to depression.

These emotional challenges are real and important.

Addressing mental health improves overall well-being.

Sleep Problems – When Rest Is Not Restful

Many COPD patients do not sleep well.

Reasons include:

Breathlessness at night

Low oxygen levels

Associated sleep apnea

Poor sleep leads to:

Daytime fatigue

Reduced concentration

Lower quality of life

Improving sleep can make a significant difference.

Pulmonary Hypertension – Increased Pressure in Lung Circulation

In advanced COPD, the blood vessels in the lungs may become affected.

This can lead to pulmonary hypertension.

It:

Increases strain on the heart

Worsens breathlessness

Reduces exercise capacity

Recognizing this condition helps guide treatment.

Increased Risk of Infections

COPD makes the lungs more vulnerable to infections.

Patients may experience:

Frequent colds

Bronchitis

Pneumonia

Each infection can worsen lung function.

Preventive measures such as vaccinations are very important.

When Multiple Conditions Exist Together

In real life, patients often have more than one condition.

For example:

COPD with heart disease

COPD with diabetes

COPD with anxiety

These combinations make management more complex.

Treatment must address all conditions together.

A Practical Example

I remember a patient who came to me with worsening breathlessness.

At first, it seemed like progression of COPD.

But further evaluation revealed heart failure.

After treating his heart condition:

His breathing improved

His energy returned

This case highlights an important point.

Not all symptoms are due to the lungs alone.

Why a Whole-Body Approach Works Better

Treating COPD effectively requires a broader perspective.

We must:

Manage the lungs

Address other health conditions

Support physical and emotional well-being

This comprehensive approach leads to better outcomes.

What This Means for You

As a patient, it is important to think beyond breathing.

Ask yourself:

How is my overall health

Am I staying active

Am I taking care of my mental well-being

This broader awareness helps you manage your condition more effectively.

Chapter Summary

COPD affects more than just the lungs

Heart disease is a common associated condition

Muscle weakness reduces physical function

Osteoporosis increases fracture risk

Weight changes can worsen symptoms

Anxiety and depression are common

Sleep problems affect overall health

Pulmonary hypertension may develop in advanced cases

Infections are more frequent

A whole-body approach improves outcomes

Action Plan for You

Focus on overall health
Do not limit attention to lungs alone

Stay physically active
Maintain muscle strength

Monitor weight and nutrition
Aim for balance

Address emotional health
Seek support if needed

Maintain regular follow-ups
Detect and manage associated conditions early

Transition to Next Chapter

Now that you understand how COPD affects the whole body, the next step is to learn how to live with it day to day. In the next chapter, we will focus on practical strategies to help you manage daily activities, conserve energy, and maintain independence

CHAPTER 15: Living with COPD – Practical Day-to-Day Strategies

Life Does Not Stop with COPD

When patients are diagnosed with COPD, one of their biggest fears is this:

"Will I be able to live a normal life?"

It is an honest concern.

The answer is not a simple yes or no.

COPD does bring limitations. But with the right approach, many patients continue to live active, meaningful, and independent lives.

This chapter is about how to do that.

Not in theory, but in real, everyday life.

Planning Your Day – A Simple but Powerful Habit

One of the most effective strategies is planning.

Instead of doing everything at once:

Spread your activities throughout the day

Do important tasks when your energy is highest

Allow time for rest

This prevents exhaustion and helps you accomplish more.

Small adjustments in planning can make a big difference.

Pacing Yourself – Finding the Right Balance

Many patients fall into two extremes.

They either:

Push themselves too hard

Avoid activity completely

Both approaches create problems.

Pacing is the balance between the two.

It means:

Moving at a steady, comfortable speed

Taking breaks before you become too breathless

Resuming activity after short rest

Over time, pacing improves endurance and confidence.

Energy Conservation – Working Smarter, Not Harder

COPD makes even simple tasks feel demanding.

Energy conservation helps you do more with less effort.

Practical tips include:

Sit while performing tasks when possible

Keep frequently used items within easy reach

Break tasks into smaller steps

Avoid unnecessary movement

These changes reduce strain and improve efficiency.

Making Your Home COPD-Friendly

Your home environment can either help or worsen your symptoms.

Simple changes can make a big difference:

Ensure good ventilation

Reduce dust and smoke exposure

Avoid strong chemical odors

Maintain comfortable temperature

A clean, organized environment supports easier breathing.

Managing Breathlessness During Daily Activities

Breathlessness is often most noticeable during routine tasks.

Here are some helpful strategies:

Use pursed-lip breathing while moving

Exhale during effort (for example, while lifting)

Move slowly and steadily

Avoid rushing

These techniques reduce the feeling of breathlessness.

Daily Activities – Making Them Easier

Let us look at some common activities.

Bathing and Dressing

Sit while bathing if needed

Take your time

Avoid rushing

Cooking

Prepare ingredients in advance

Use simple cooking methods

Sit when possible

Walking

Walk at a comfortable pace

Take breaks when needed

Use support if required

The goal is not to avoid these activities, but to adapt them.

Staying Social – Do Not Withdraw

One of the silent problems in COPD is social isolation.

Patients may avoid:

Social gatherings

Visiting friends

Public places

This often happens due to fear of breathlessness.

But isolation leads to:

Reduced emotional well-being

Increased anxiety

Staying connected is important.

Even small interactions make a difference.

Managing Anxiety During Breathlessness

Breathlessness can create anxiety. Anxiety can worsen breathing.

This creates a cycle.

To break this cycle:

Sit down and relax your shoulders

Focus on slow breathing

Use pursed-lip breathing

Understanding that breathlessness can be managed reduces fear.

Maintaining Independence

Independence is closely linked to confidence.

COPD may slow you down, but it does not take away your ability to function.

With proper strategies:

You can manage daily tasks

You can maintain self-confidence

You can stay independent

Accept help when needed, but continue doing what you can.

Traveling with COPD – It Is Possible

Many patients assume they cannot travel.

That is not true.

With planning:

Carry your medications

Arrange oxygen if needed

Plan rest breaks

Travel may require more preparation, but it remains possible.

The Role of Family Support

Family support plays an important role.

They can help with:

Encouragement

Assistance with tasks

Emotional support

At the same time, balance is important.

Too much dependence reduces confidence. Too little support increases stress.

Communication helps maintain the right balance.

A Practical Example

I remember a patient who gradually stopped going out.

He became less active and more withdrawn.

We worked on small changes:

Short walks

Simple daily routines

Reconnecting with friends

Over time:

His activity increased

His confidence improved

His outlook became more positive

His lung function had not changed significantly. But his life had improved.

Why Attitude Matters

Living with COPD is not only physical. It is also mental.

Patients who:

Stay engaged

Remain active

Adapt to limitations

often do better than those who withdraw.

This is not about ignoring the disease.

It is about learning to live with it effectively.

What This Means for You

COPD may require adjustments.

But it does not mean giving up your life.

With thoughtful changes, you can:

Stay active

Remain independent

Maintain quality of life

Chapter Summary

COPD does not mean the end of an active life

Planning and pacing help conserve energy

Energy conservation improves efficiency

A supportive home environment helps breathing

Breathing techniques reduce symptoms

Daily activities can be adapted

Social interaction is important

Anxiety can be managed with simple techniques

Independence can be maintained

A positive approach improves outcomes

Action Plan for You

Plan your daily activities
Spread tasks throughout the day

Practice pacing
Avoid overexertion

Use energy conservation techniques
Reduce unnecessary effort

Stay socially connected
Avoid isolation

Use breathing techniques
Manage breathlessness

Transition to Next Chapter

Now that you understand how to manage daily life with COPD, the next step is to focus on lifestyle factors in more detail. In the next chapter, we will discuss diet, exercise, and healthy living in a deeper and more structured way.

CHAPTER 16: Diet, Exercise, and Healthy Living – Building Strength from Within

Why Lifestyle Is a Powerful Treatment

When patients think about COPD treatment, they usually think about inhalers.

But there is another side to treatment that is just as important.

What you eat.
How you move.
How you live every day.

I have seen patients with similar lung function do very differently. The difference often lies in lifestyle.

The body has a remarkable ability to adapt. When you support it properly, it responds.

This chapter is about using that ability.

Nutrition – Fueling Your Body for Better Breathing

Breathing in COPD requires more effort than normal.

That means your body uses more energy.

At the same time, many patients experience:

Reduced appetite

Fatigue while eating

Weight changes

This creates a challenge.

Some patients lose weight and become weak. Others gain weight and become less active.

Both situations can worsen symptoms.

If You Are Losing Weight – Rebuilding Strength

Weight loss in COPD is not just about appearance.

It often reflects loss of muscle mass.

This leads to:

Reduced strength

Lower energy

Increased breathlessness

If you are underweight:

Eat small, frequent meals

Focus on protein-rich foods

Add calorie-dense foods

Rest before meals

The goal is to rebuild strength gradually.

If You Are Overweight – Reducing the Burden

Excess weight increases the effort required to breathe.

It:

Limits movement

Increases fatigue

Worsens breathlessness

Gradual weight reduction can help.

Focus on:

Balanced meals

Portion control

Regular activity

Avoid crash diets. Slow, steady progress works best.

Eating Smart – Simple Practical Tips

Small changes can make eating easier:

Eat slowly and chew well

Avoid large, heavy meals

Choose easy-to-digest foods

Stay well hydrated

Some patients feel more breathless after large meals.

Smaller portions help prevent this.

Exercise – The Most Effective Habit You Can Build

Exercise is one of the most powerful tools in COPD care.

It may feel difficult at first.

But over time, it becomes easier.

Benefits include:

Improved muscle strength

Better endurance

Reduced breathlessness

Increased confidence

The key is consistency.

Types of Exercise That Work Best

You do not need complicated routines.

Simple activities are enough.

Walking

The easiest and most practical exercise

Can be done anywhere

Living with COPD: Daily Tips for Better Management

Managing COPD involves making lifestyle changes that can help improve the quality of life and reduce symptoms. Here are key daily tips for living with COPD:

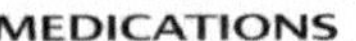

MEDICATIONS

- ✓ Take medications as prescribed
- ✓ Keep an inhaler with you for quick relief.

OXYGEN THERAPY

- ✓ Use oxygen prescribed
- ✓ Ensure equipment is leared and used safely.

Lungs (COPD)

HEALTHY EATING

- ✓ Muscle weakness
- ✓ Reduced exercise tolerance.

AVOID TRIGGERS

- ✓ Osteoporosis risk
- ✓ Fracture risk.

MOOD / MENTAL HEALTH

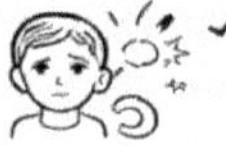

- ✓ Attend regular check-ups.

PHYSICAL ACTIVITY

- ✓ Engage in regular, moderate exercise.

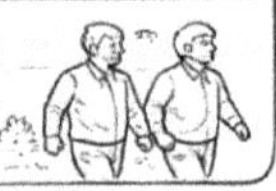

WORK CLOSELY WITH YOUR DOCTOR

- ✓ Attend regular check-ups.
- ✓ Discuss any changes in symptoms or concerns.

Strength Training

Light weights or resistance bands

Helps maintain muscle mass

Stretching

Improves flexibility

Reduces stiffness

A combination of these gives the best results.

How to Exercise Safely

Safety is important.

Start slowly

Warm up before activity

Use breathing techniques

Stop if you feel severe discomfort

Keep your inhaler nearby

Remember, progress is gradual.

Breaking the Cycle of Inactivity

Many patients avoid exercise because they fear breathlessness.

This is understandable.

But avoiding activity leads to:

Weak muscles

Reduced stamina

Increased breathlessness

Exercise helps break this cycle.

Building a Routine That Lasts

Consistency matters more than intensity.

A simple routine might include:

Daily walking

Light strength exercises a few times per week

Over time, this becomes a habit.

Sleep – Restoring Energy

Good sleep is essential for overall health.

Poor sleep leads to:

Fatigue

Reduced concentration

Irritability

To improve sleep:

Maintain a regular schedule

Avoid heavy meals before bedtime

Create a comfortable sleep environment

If sleep problems persist, discuss them with your doctor.

Stress and Breathing – A Close Connection

Stress affects breathing.

When you are anxious:

Breathing becomes rapid and shallow

Muscles become tense

Breathlessness increases

Managing stress helps improve breathing.

Simple strategies include:

Slow breathing exercises

Relaxation techniques

Engaging in enjoyable activities

Healthy Habits That Support Your Lungs

In addition to diet and exercise:

Avoid smoking and pollutants

Stay up to date with vaccinations

Maintain regular medical follow-up

These habits support long-term health.

A Practical Example

I remember a patient who felt constantly tired and breathless.

His lifestyle was very sedentary, and his eating pattern was irregular.

We made simple changes:

Daily walking

Balanced meals

Better sleep routine

Over time:

His energy improved

His breathlessness reduced

His confidence returned

These changes were simple, but powerful.

Why Small Changes Matter

You do not need to change everything at once.

Small steps lead to meaningful results.

A short walk

A balanced meal

A good night's sleep

These simple habits build strength over time.

What This Means for You

Lifestyle is not an optional part of treatment.

It is a central part.

By focusing on:

Nutrition

Exercise

Healthy habits

you can improve your quality of life significantly.

Chapter Summary

Lifestyle plays a major role in COPD management

Proper nutrition supports strength and energy

Both weight loss and weight gain can worsen symptoms

Exercise improves stamina and reduces breathlessness

Walking, strength training, and stretching are effective

Consistency is more important than intensity

Sleep and stress management are important

Small changes lead to meaningful improvements

Action Plan for You

Review your diet
Aim for balanced nutrition

Start regular exercise
Begin with simple activities

Build a routine
Consistency is key

Focus on sleep and stress
Support overall health

Take small steps
Gradual progress leads to lasting results

Transition to Next Chapter

Now that you understand the role of lifestyle, the next step is to look at how COPD behaves in different people. In the next chapter, we will discuss special situations and how COPD varies from person to person.

CHAPTER 17: COPD in Special Situations – Why Every Patient Is Different

One Disease, Many Different Experiences

One of the most important lessons I have learned in medicine is this:

No two patients are exactly alike.

COPD may have a common name, but it does not behave the same way in everyone.

Two patients may have:

Similar test results

Similar exposure history

Yet their symptoms, progression, and response to treatment can be very different.

Understanding these variations helps us provide better, more personalized care.

COPD in Women – Often Underrecognized

For many years, COPD was considered mainly a disease of men.

That is no longer true.

More women are now affected, and in some cases, the disease behaves differently.

Women may:

Develop symptoms with less smoking exposure

Experience more breathlessness

Be diagnosed later because symptoms are underestimated

Hormonal and biological differences may play a role.

The key message is simple.

COPD in women should be recognized early and treated with the same seriousness.

COPD in Younger Patients – When It Appears Early

COPD is usually diagnosed after the age of 40.

But in some cases, it appears earlier.

Possible reasons include:

Genetic conditions

Early and heavy exposure to smoking or pollution

Poor lung development during childhood

When COPD develops early:

Progression may be more significant over time

Early intervention becomes even more important

Identifying the cause is essential.

COPD in Non-Smokers – A Common Misunderstanding

Many people believe COPD occurs only in smokers.

This is not correct.

A significant number of patients with COPD have never smoked.

Common causes include:

Indoor pollution

Occupational exposure

Environmental pollutants

Past lung infections

This is important because it changes how we think about risk.

If symptoms are present, COPD should be considered, even in non-smokers.

Genetic COPD – When the Risk Is Inherited

In some patients, genetics play a role.

The most well-known example is **alpha-1 antitrypsin deficiency**.

In these patients:

Lung damage can occur at a younger age

Disease may progress faster

Identifying this condition is important because:

It influences treatment

Family members may need screening

Occupational Exposure – The Workplace Factor

Many patients do not realize that their job may have contributed to their condition.

Long-term exposure to:

Dust

Chemicals

Fumes

can damage the lungs.

Common high-risk occupations include:

Construction

Mining

Factory work

Agriculture

Reducing exposure moving forward is essential.

COPD in Older Adults – Balancing Care

COPD is most common in older adults.

In this group:

Multiple health conditions often coexist

Physical strength may be reduced

Recovery from illness may take longer

Treatment needs to be balanced carefully.

The goal is:

Symptom relief

Maintaining independence

Minimizing side effects

Asthma and COPD Overlap – A Unique Situation

Some patients have features of both asthma and COPD.

They may:

Have a history of asthma

Show partial improvement with bronchodilators

Experience variable symptoms

These patients require a tailored approach.

Treatment may differ from typical COPD management.

Environmental and Lifestyle Influences

Even after diagnosis, environment continues to matter.

Factors such as:

Air quality

Smoking exposure

Physical activity

Nutrition

affect how COPD progresses.

Improving these factors helps improve outcomes.

A Practical Example

I remember two patients with similar symptoms.

One was a smoker. The other had never smoked but worked for years in a dusty environment.

Both had COPD.

This highlights an important point.

The cause may differ, but the impact on the lungs can be similar.

Why Personalized Care Matters

Because COPD varies so much, treatment must be individualized.

A one-size-fits-all approach does not work.

Care should be tailored based on:

Risk factors

Severity

Lifestyle

Patient goals

This approach leads to better outcomes.

What This Means for You

Your COPD is your own.

It is shaped by your:

History

Lifestyle

Health conditions

Understanding your specific situation helps you take better control.

Chapter Summary

COPD varies significantly between individuals

Women may experience different patterns

COPD can occur in younger patients

Non-smokers can develop COPD

Genetic factors may play a role

Occupational exposure is important

Older adults require balanced care

Asthma-COPD overlap needs special attention

Environmental factors continue to influence the disease

Personalized care improves outcomes

Action Plan for You

Understand your personal risk factors
Identify what applies to you

Discuss your individual situation with your doctor
Tailored care is more effective

Reduce harmful exposures
Protect your lungs

Stay informed
Knowledge improves control

Focus on what you can change
Small steps matter

Transition to Next Chapter

Now that you understand how COPD varies from person to person, the next step is to focus on prevention and early detection. In the next chapter, we will discuss how to protect lung health and reduce the risk of progression

CHAPTER 18: Prevention and Early Detection – Protecting Your Lungs Before It Is Too Late

Why Prevention Is Always Better Than Treatment

After understanding COPD in depth, it is natural to ask:

"Could this have been prevented?"

In many cases, the answer is yes.

COPD usually develops slowly over many years. This gives us a valuable opportunity.

If we recognize the risks early and take the right steps, we can:

Reduce the chances of developing COPD

Slow its progression

Preserve lung function

Prevention is not complicated. But it requires awareness and action.

Who Is at Risk

The first step in prevention is knowing who is at risk.

You may be at higher risk if you:

Smoke or have smoked in the past

Are exposed to secondhand smoke

Work in dusty or chemical environments

Live in areas with poor air quality

Have a family history of lung disease

Had frequent lung infections in childhood

If any of these apply, it is important to be proactive.

Recognizing Early Warning Signs

COPD does not start suddenly.

Early symptoms are often mild and easy to ignore.

These may include:

Mild breathlessness during activity

Occasional cough

Reduced stamina

Frequent respiratory infections

These are early signals.

Ignoring them allows the disease to progress.

Recognizing them early creates an opportunity to act.

The Role of Early Evaluation

Unlike some diseases, COPD is not routinely screened in everyone.

But targeted evaluation is very important.

This means:

Identifying individuals with risk factors

Testing them even if symptoms are mild

Simple tools such as:

Questionnaires

Spirometry

can detect early disease.

Early detection changes outcomes.

Smoking – The Most Important Preventable Cause

The most effective way to prevent COPD is to avoid smoking.

If you do not smoke, do not start.

If you smoke, quitting is the single most important step you can take.

It helps at every stage:

Before symptoms develop

After early symptoms

Even after diagnosis

Stopping smoking slows disease progression significantly.

Reducing Environmental Exposure

Protecting your lungs from harmful exposures is essential.

At home:

Ensure good ventilation

Avoid indoor smoke

Use cleaner fuels when possible

At work:

Use protective equipment

Follow safety guidelines

Reduce exposure to dust and chemicals

Small changes can have a lasting impact.

Protecting Lung Health Early in Life

Lung health begins in childhood.

Factors that influence long-term lung function include:

Nutrition

Exposure to smoke

Respiratory infections

Protecting children from harmful exposures helps reduce future risk.

Vaccinations – A Simple Preventive Step

Vaccinations are an important part of prevention.

They reduce:

Respiratory infections

Risk of complications

Frequency of flare-ups

Important vaccines include:

Influenza

Pneumococcal

COVID-19

These are especially important for at-risk individuals.

Healthy Lifestyle – Supporting Lung Function

A healthy lifestyle supports overall lung health.

This includes:

Regular physical activity

Balanced nutrition

Avoiding harmful exposures

Managing stress

These habits strengthen the body and improve resilience.

Why COPD Is Often Diagnosed Late

Despite available tools, COPD is often diagnosed late.

Common reasons include:

Ignoring early symptoms

Lack of awareness

Limited use of spirometry

Assuming symptoms are due to aging

Improving awareness is key.

A Practical Example

I remember a patient who came for a routine check-up.

He mentioned mild breathlessness but did not consider it important.

Because of his smoking history, we performed spirometry.

The test showed early COPD.

He quit smoking and made lifestyle changes.

Years later, his condition remained stable.

That is the power of early detection.

Prevention Is a Shared Responsibility

Preventing COPD is not only an individual effort.

It also depends on:

Public health awareness

Workplace safety

Environmental protection

When these factors come together, the impact is much greater.

What This Means for You

Whether you already have COPD or are at risk, this chapter carries an important message.

You have the ability to influence your lung health.

Small actions taken early can prevent larger problems later.

Chapter Summary

COPD can often be prevented or delayed

Recognizing risk factors is essential

Early symptoms should not be ignored

Targeted evaluation helps detect disease early

Smoking cessation is the most important step

Reducing environmental exposure protects lung health

Childhood factors influence future risk

Vaccinations reduce infections and complications

Healthy lifestyle supports lung function

Early detection improves long-term outcomes

Action Plan for You

Identify your risk factors
Be aware of exposures and habits

Take early symptoms seriously
Do not ignore mild changes

Quit smoking or avoid it completely
This is the most important step

Protect your environment
Reduce exposure to pollutants

Seek early evaluation
Testing can detect disease early

Transition to Next Chapter

Now that we have discussed prevention and early detection, the next step is to understand advanced COPD and how care shifts in later stages. In the next chapter, we will focus on comfort, planning, and maintaining dignity when the disease becomes more severe.

CHAPTER 19: Advanced COPD – Comfort, Planning, and Preserving Dignity

When COPD Reaches an Advanced Stage

As COPD progresses, the challenges change.

In earlier stages, the focus is on controlling symptoms and staying active.

In advanced COPD, the focus becomes broader:

Managing persistent symptoms

Maintaining comfort

Preserving independence and dignity

This stage requires a different kind of attention.

Not just medical treatment, but thoughtful, compassionate care.

What Advanced COPD Feels Like

Patients with advanced COPD often experience:

Breathlessness with minimal activity or even at rest

Frequent flare-ups

Reduced ability to perform daily tasks

Increased fatigue

Simple activities may become difficult.

This can be frustrating and emotionally challenging.

The Goal of Care Changes

At this stage, the goal is not only to treat the disease.

The goal is to improve quality of life.

This includes:

Reducing discomfort

Supporting daily functioning

Minimizing hospital visits

Providing emotional support

Care becomes more personalized and focused on comfort.

Managing Breathlessness – The Central Focus

Breathlessness remains the most distressing symptom.

Management includes:

Optimizing inhaler therapy

Using oxygen when needed

Practicing breathing techniques

Using medications to reduce discomfort

Sometimes, additional medications are used carefully to relieve severe breathlessness.

The aim is always to improve comfort.

Energy Conservation Becomes Essential

At this stage, conserving energy is very important.

Patients are encouraged to:

Prioritize essential activities

Take frequent rest breaks

Use assistive devices if needed

This helps maintain independence while reducing exhaustion.

Nutrition and Strength – Preventing Further Decline

Advanced COPD often leads to weight loss and muscle weakness.

Maintaining nutrition helps:

Preserve strength

Improve energy

Support overall health

Small, frequent meals are often easier to manage.

Emotional Support – A Key Part of Care

Living with advanced COPD can be emotionally overwhelming.

Patients may feel:

Anxiety about breathing

Fear of flare-ups

Concern about the future

Support from:

Family

Healthcare providers

Counselors

can make a significant difference.

Palliative Care – Improving Quality of Life

The term "palliative care" is often misunderstood.

It does not mean giving up.

It means focusing on:

Comfort

Symptom relief

Emotional support

Palliative care can be introduced at any stage, but it becomes especially important in advanced disease.

It works alongside other treatments.

Planning Ahead – A Thoughtful Approach

One of the most important aspects of advanced care is planning.

This includes:

Discussing treatment preferences

Deciding how aggressive care should be

Identifying emergency plans

These discussions are not easy, but they provide clarity.

They help ensure that care aligns with the patient's wishes.

Advanced Directives – Making Your Wishes Known

Advanced directives allow patients to express their preferences.

This may include:

Hospital care decisions

Use of life-support measures

Preferred place of care

Having these decisions documented reduces uncertainty during emergencies.

Supporting the Family

COPD affects not only the patient, but also the family.

Family members often:

Provide daily support

Share emotional stress

Help with decision-making

Including them in discussions improves care and reduces confusion.

Avoiding Unnecessary Hospitalizations

Frequent hospital visits can be stressful.

With proper planning:

Many flare-ups can be managed early

Home-based care can be optimized

The goal is to reduce unnecessary hospital stays while ensuring safety.

Maintaining Dignity and Independence

Even in advanced stages, dignity remains central.

This includes:

Respecting patient preferences

Supporting independence as much as possible

Providing compassionate care

Dignity is not dependent on physical ability.

It comes from how care is delivered.

A Practical Example

I remember a patient with advanced COPD who feared losing control over his life.

We discussed his preferences openly.

We created a clear plan.

Over time:

He felt more secure

His anxiety reduced

His family felt more prepared

The disease had not changed significantly.

But his sense of control had improved.

Why This Stage Requires a Different Perspective

Advanced COPD is not just about managing symptoms.

It is about:

Living with comfort

Maintaining dignity

Supporting emotional well-being

This requires a thoughtful and compassionate approach.

What This Means for You

If you or your loved one is dealing with advanced COPD:

Focus on:

Comfort

Clear communication

Support systems

You are not alone in this journey.

Chapter Summary

Advanced COPD brings new challenges

The focus shifts toward comfort and quality of life

Breathlessness management becomes central

Energy conservation is essential

Nutrition supports strength

Emotional support is important

Palliative care improves quality of life

Planning ahead provides clarity

Family support plays a key role

Dignity must always be preserved

Action Plan for You

Focus on comfort
Prioritize what matters most

Discuss your preferences
Plan ahead with your doctor

Use available support
Involve family and caregivers

Manage symptoms actively
Do not ignore discomfort

Maintain dignity and independence
Stay engaged in your care

Transition to Next Chapter

Now that we have discussed advanced COPD, the next step is to address common questions patients often have. In the next chapter, we will answer frequently asked questions to clear doubts and provide practical clarity.

CHAPTER 20: Frequently Asked Questions – Clear, Honest Answers

Why Questions Matter in COPD

In my experience, patients often carry many questions, but they do not always ask them.

Sometimes they feel the question is too simple. Sometimes they hesitate. Sometimes they accept uncertainty.

But unanswered questions create anxiety.

This chapter is meant to address the most common and important questions I hear in daily practice.

Clear answers bring clarity. And clarity builds confidence.

Can COPD Be Cured?

This is the most common question.

The honest answer is no.

COPD cannot be completely cured because the damage to the lungs cannot be fully reversed.

But this is not the full story.

COPD can be managed effectively.

With proper care:

Symptoms can improve

Progression can slow

Quality of life can remain good

Many patients live active and meaningful lives with COPD.

Will My Breathing Keep Getting Worse?

Not necessarily.

COPD is a progressive condition, but the rate of progression varies.

If you:

Quit smoking

Use medications regularly

Stay active

you can slow the decline significantly.

Some patients remain stable for many years.

Can I Exercise Safely?

Yes. In fact, you should.

Exercise:

Improves strength

Increases endurance

Reduces breathlessness over time

Start slowly and increase gradually.

Avoiding exercise actually worsens symptoms.

Is Breathlessness Just Part of Aging?

No.

Mild changes in stamina may occur with age, but significant breathlessness is not normal.

If you feel limited due to breathing, it needs evaluation.

Will I Need Oxygen Therapy?

Not every patient requires oxygen.

Oxygen is prescribed only when levels are low.

Some patients may never need it. Others may need it during activity or sleep.

When used appropriately, it improves comfort and health.

Are Inhalers Addictive?

No.

This is a common misconception.

Inhalers are not addictive. They are essential medications that help your lungs function better.

Using them regularly is beneficial.

What Should I Do If My Symptoms Suddenly Worsen?

This may be a flare-up.

You should:

Use your rescue inhaler

Follow your action plan

Monitor symptoms

Seek medical help if symptoms do not improve or become severe.

Early action is very important.

Can I Travel with COPD?

Yes, with proper planning.

Carry your medications

Plan for oxygen if needed

Avoid exposure to poor air quality

Many patients travel successfully with COPD.

How Long Can I Live with COPD?

This depends on several factors:

Severity of the disease

Smoking status

Overall health

Frequency of flare-ups

With proper care, many patients live for many years.

The focus should be on living well.

Can COPD Affect My Heart?

Yes.

COPD and heart disease often occur together.

Low oxygen levels and lung changes can strain the heart.

Managing both conditions is important.

Why Do I Feel Anxious When I Am Breathless?

This is very common.

Breathlessness can trigger anxiety, and anxiety can worsen breathing.

Learning breathing techniques and staying calm can help break this cycle.

Can Diet Make a Difference?

Yes.

Good nutrition:

Supports energy

Maintains strength

Helps manage weight

Both underweight and overweight can worsen symptoms.

Do I Need to Take Medicines Even When I Feel Fine?

Yes.

Many COPD medications are preventive.

Stopping them when you feel better can lead to worsening symptoms.

Consistency is essential.

Is It Safe to Continue Working?

In many cases, yes.

This depends on:

Severity of symptoms

Type of work

Exposure to dust or chemicals

With adjustments, many patients continue to work.

Can I Prevent COPD from Getting Worse?

Yes, to a large extent.

Key steps include:

Quitting smoking

Taking medications regularly

Staying active

Avoiding triggers

Preventing infections

These actions can significantly slow progression.

A Practical Example

I remember a patient who came with many concerns.

He was afraid to exercise, travel, or even go out.

We addressed his questions one by one.

Over time:

His confidence improved

His activity increased

His quality of life improved

Sometimes, the biggest barrier is uncertainty.

Why Asking Questions Is Important

Never hesitate to ask.

Good communication with your doctor:

Improves understanding

Builds trust

Leads to better care

There are no small questions when it comes to your health.

Chapter Summary

COPD cannot be cured but can be managed effectively

Disease progression can be slowed

Exercise is safe and beneficial

Breathlessness is not a normal part of aging

Oxygen therapy is used when needed

Inhalers are safe and not addictive

Flare-ups require early action

Travel and work are often possible

Anxiety is common and manageable

Diet and lifestyle play important roles

Action Plan for You

Ask questions openly
Clarity improves confidence

Follow your treatment plan
Consistency is essential

Stay active
Do not limit yourself unnecessarily

Manage anxiety
Use breathing techniques

Focus on long-term health
Small daily actions matter

Transition to Next Chapter

Now that we have answered the most common questions, the next step is to clear common myths about COPD. In the next chapter, we will address misconceptions that often create confusion and delay proper care.

CHAPTER 21: Common Myths About COPD – Clearing Misconceptions

Why Myths Can Mislead You

Over the years, I have realized that many patients do not struggle only with COPD.

They also struggle with misinformation.

Some of these beliefs are passed from others. Some come from incomplete understanding. Some come from fear.

The problem is simple.

When myths replace facts:

Diagnosis is delayed

Treatment is not followed properly

Anxiety increases

This chapter is about replacing confusion with clarity.

Myth 1: "COPD Happens Only to Smokers"

This is one of the most common myths.

Smoking is the leading cause, but it is not the only cause.

COPD can also occur due to:

Indoor pollution

Occupational exposure

Environmental factors

Genetic conditions

I have treated many patients who never smoked.

The truth is clear.

Smoking increases risk, but it is not the only reason.

Myth 2: "Breathlessness Is Just Part of Aging"

Many patients ignore symptoms because of this belief.

But significant breathlessness is not normal.

If you:

Avoid activities due to breathing

Feel limited in daily tasks

it needs evaluation.

Ignoring symptoms delays diagnosis.

Myth 3: "Nothing Can Be Done Once You Have COPD"

This is not true.

While COPD cannot be cured, it can be managed effectively.

Treatment can:

Improve symptoms

Reduce flare-ups

Slow progression

Improve quality of life

Many patients live well with proper care.

Myth 4: “Inhalers Are Addictive”

This is a common concern.

Inhalers are not addictive.

They are essential medications that help:

Open airways

Reduce inflammation

Improve breathing

Avoiding them due to fear can worsen symptoms.

Myth 5: “Oxygen Means the End Stage”

Many patients fear oxygen therapy.

They feel it signals the end of their condition.

This is not correct.

Oxygen is used when the body needs support.

It helps:

Improve energy

Protect vital organs

Improve quality of life

It is a tool, not a failure.

Myth 6: "Exercise Will Make Things Worse"

This belief leads to inactivity.

In reality, exercise:

Improves strength

Increases endurance

Reduces breathlessness over time

Avoiding activity makes symptoms worse.

Exercise should be done gradually and safely.

Myth 7: "If I Feel Fine, I Do Not Need Treatment"

Many patients stop medications when they feel better.

This leads to:

Loss of symptom control

Increased flare-ups

COPD treatment is preventive.

Regular use is important, even when you feel well.

Myth 8: "Only Severe Symptoms Need Attention"

COPD often begins with mild symptoms.

Waiting for severe symptoms:

Delays diagnosis

Allows progression

Early attention leads to better outcomes.

Myth 9: "COPD Means I Cannot Live Normally"

This is one of the most discouraging myths.

COPD does bring challenges.

But with proper management:

Many patients remain active

Continue social activities

Maintain independence

The goal is to live well, not just manage disease.

Why These Myths Continue

These myths persist because:

Awareness is limited

Symptoms are misunderstood

Information is often incomplete

This is why education is so important.

A Practical Example

I remember a patient who avoided inhalers for months because he believed they were harmful.

His symptoms worsened.

Once he understood the facts and started treatment:

His breathing improved

His activity increased

His confidence returned

Correct information changed his outcome.

Replacing Fear with Knowledge

Fear often comes from uncertainty.

When you understand your condition:

You feel more in control

You make better decisions

You follow treatment confidently

Knowledge reduces fear.

What This Means for You

Do not accept information without questioning it.

If something does not seem right:

Ask your doctor

Seek reliable sources

Your decisions should be based on facts, not myths.

Chapter Summary

Myths about COPD can delay diagnosis and treatment

COPD is not limited to smokers

Breathlessness is not a normal part of aging

COPD can be managed effectively

Inhalers are safe and not addictive

Oxygen therapy is supportive, not a sign of failure

Exercise is beneficial and necessary

Regular treatment is essential

Patients can live active and meaningful lives

Action Plan for You

Identify misconceptions
Recognize incorrect beliefs

Seek accurate information
Rely on trusted sources

Follow evidence-based treatment
Trust your doctor's guidance

Stay active and engaged
Do not limit yourself unnecessarily

Ask questions
Clarify doubts early

Transition to Next Chapter

Now that we have cleared common myths, the next step is to bring everything together into a practical, personalized plan. In the next chapter, we will help you create your own COPD management plan for daily life.

CHAPTER 22: Creating Your Personal COPD Plan – A Clear Path Forward

Why You Need a Personal Plan

By now, you have learned a great deal about COPD.

But knowledge alone is not enough.

What truly makes a difference is how you apply this knowledge to your daily life.

Every patient is different:

Symptoms vary

Lifestyle differs

Goals are personal

That is why a one-size-fits-all approach does not work.

A personal plan gives you:

Structure

Clarity

Confidence

It turns information into action.

Step 1: Know Your Baseline

The first step is understanding your normal.

Ask yourself:

How far can I walk comfortably

What activities can I perform easily

How breathless do I feel on a typical day

This becomes your baseline.

Once you know this, you can quickly recognize changes.

Step 2: Identify Your Symptoms Clearly

Be specific about your symptoms.

Track:

Breathlessness

Cough

Sputum

Energy level

Writing these down helps you:

Notice patterns

Detect early changes

Communicate better with your doctor

Step 3: Understand Your Medications

Your treatment plan should be clear.

Know:

Which inhalers are for daily use

Which inhalers are for quick relief

When and how to use each

This avoids confusion and improves effectiveness.

Step 4: Create a Flare-Up Action Plan

Every patient should have a clear plan for worsening symptoms.

Your plan should include:

Early warning signs

What medications to use

When to contact your doctor

When to seek emergency care

This reduces panic and helps you act quickly.

Step 5: Build a Daily Routine

A structured routine improves consistency.

Include:

Fixed medication times

Planned physical activity

Rest periods

Avoid trying to do everything at once.

Steady routines reduce stress and improve control.

Step 6: Stay Physically Active

Activity is essential.

Choose what works for you:

Walking

Light exercises

Breathing exercises

Start small and increase gradually.

Consistency matters more than intensity.

Step 7: Focus on Nutrition

Your plan should include simple dietary goals.

Depending on your situation:

Maintain a healthy weight

Eat balanced meals

Avoid heavy meals

Good nutrition supports strength and energy.

Step 8: Reduce Risk Factors

Identify what worsens your symptoms.

This may include:

Smoking

Pollution

Dust or chemicals

Take steps to reduce exposure.

This protects your lungs.

Step 9: Monitor Your Progress

Regular monitoring keeps you on track.

You can:

Track symptoms

Note changes in activity

Record flare-ups

This helps you act early.

Step 10: Plan Regular Follow-Ups

Your plan should include regular visits with your doctor.

These visits help:

Adjust treatment

Monitor progression

Address concerns

Do not wait for symptoms to worsen.

Step 11: Be Prepared for Emergencies

Preparation reduces fear.

Know:

When symptoms are serious

Where to seek help

Which medications to carry

This ensures timely action.

Step 12: Support Your Mental Well-Being

Your plan should include emotional health.

Living with COPD can be stressful.

Focus on:

Staying engaged

Maintaining social connections

Managing anxiety

Mental strength supports physical health.

A Simple Example of a Personal Plan

Let me give you a simple example.

A patient's plan may include:

Morning inhaler use

Daily walking for 15 minutes

Afternoon rest

Monitoring symptoms

Using rescue inhaler if needed

Contacting doctor if symptoms worsen

This is simple, but effective.

Why Personal Plans Work

Patients with a clear plan:

Feel more confident

Act earlier

Experience fewer complications

Without a plan, patients often feel uncertain.

Taking Ownership of Your Health

Your plan is not something given to you.

It is something you create with your doctor.

It reflects your:

Condition

Lifestyle

Goals

This sense of ownership makes a difference.

What This Means for You

You do not need a complicated plan.

You need a clear and practical one.

Simple, consistent actions lead to better outcomes.

Chapter Summary

A personal COPD plan provides structure and clarity

Knowing your baseline helps detect changes

Symptom tracking improves awareness

Understanding medications is essential

A flare-up plan allows early action

Daily routines improve consistency

Exercise and nutrition support health

Reducing risk factors slows progression

Regular follow-ups ensure proper care

Mental well-being is important

Action Plan for You

Write your personal plan
Keep it simple and practical

Know your baseline
Recognize your normal

Follow your treatment regularly
Consistency is key

Stay active and eat well
Support your health

Be prepared for flare-ups
Act early

Transition to Next Chapter

Now that you have a personal plan, the next step is to look ahead. In the next chapter, we will focus on long-term living with COPD, maintaining stability, and continuing to live with confidence.

CHAPTER 23: Staying Well Long-Term – Living with Stability and Confidence

The Long View of COPD

COPD is not a short-term illness.

It is a long-term condition that becomes part of your life.

At first, this realization can feel overwhelming.

But over time, many patients discover something important.

With the right approach, COPD does not have to control your life.

You can learn to live with it, manage it, and maintain stability.

This chapter is about that long-term journey.

What Does "Staying Stable" Really Mean

Stability does not mean the disease disappears.

It means:

Symptoms remain controlled

Flare-ups are infrequent

Daily activities are manageable

Overall health is maintained

Many patients achieve this level of stability.

It is a realistic and meaningful goal.

Consistency – The Most Powerful Habit

If I had to choose one factor that makes the biggest difference over time, it would be consistency.

Patients who:

Take medications regularly

Stay active

Follow their plan

tend to do much better than those who are inconsistent.

Small, daily actions matter more than occasional effort.

Preventing Flare-Ups – The Key to Long-Term Health

Flare-ups are turning points.

Each flare-up can:

Worsen lung function

Reduce confidence

Increase future risk

Preventing them is one of the most important goals.

This includes:

Taking medications regularly

Staying up to date with vaccinations

Avoiding infections

Recognizing early symptoms

Prevention protects your long-term health.

Regular Follow-Up – Staying on Track

COPD care is not a one-time decision.

It requires ongoing monitoring.

Regular visits help:

Adjust medications

Detect changes early

Address new concerns

Even when you feel well, follow-up remains important.

Adapting as Life Changes

Over time, your condition and circumstances may change.

Your plan should evolve accordingly.

For example:

Activity levels may need adjustment

Medications may change

New health conditions may develop

Flexibility is important.

What works today may need adjustment tomorrow.

Staying Active – A Lifelong Commitment

Activity is not just for short-term improvement.

It is a lifelong habit.

Even in later stages:

Gentle activity helps maintain strength

Movement prevents further decline

The goal is not perfection.

The goal is to keep moving.

Maintaining Emotional Balance

Living with a chronic condition can affect your mindset.

There may be:

Good days

Difficult days

Maintaining emotional balance helps you stay consistent.

Helpful strategies include:

Staying engaged with family and friends

Keeping a routine

Focusing on what you can do

A stable mind supports a stable body.

Building a Support System

Long-term success is rarely achieved alone.

Support may come from:

Family

Friends

Healthcare providers

Having people who understand your condition makes a difference.

Avoiding Common Pitfalls

Over time, some patients fall into patterns that worsen their condition.

Common pitfalls include:

Skipping medications

Becoming inactive

Ignoring symptoms

Delaying medical care

Recognizing these patterns early helps you stay on track.

A Practical Example

I remember a patient who initially struggled with COPD.

He had frequent flare-ups and felt discouraged.

Over time, he adopted a consistent routine:

Regular medication use

Daily walking

Early response to symptoms

Over the years:

His flare-ups reduced

His activity improved

His confidence returned

The disease did not disappear.

But his control over it improved significantly.

Why Long-Term Thinking Matters

COPD is a marathon, not a sprint.

Short-term improvements are encouraging.

But long-term stability is the real goal.

This requires:

Patience

Consistency

Adaptation

What This Means for You

You do not have to do everything perfectly.

You just have to keep moving in the right direction.

Small, steady steps lead to lasting results.

Chapter Summary

COPD requires long-term management

Stability means controlled symptoms and fewer flare-ups

Consistency is the most important factor

Preventing flare-ups protects lung function

Regular follow-up ensures proper care

Plans should adapt over time

Staying active is essential

Emotional balance supports long-term success

Support systems improve outcomes

Action Plan for You

Stay consistent with your care
Daily habits matter

Prevent flare-ups
Focus on early action

Attend regular follow-ups
Stay connected with your doctor

Keep moving
Maintain physical activity

Stay positive and engaged
Focus on what you can control

Transition to Next Chapter

Now that we have discussed long-term stability, the next and final chapter will bring everything together. We will focus on living with confidence, maintaining hope, and moving forward despite COPD.

CHAPTER 24: Moving Forward with Confidence – Living Fully with COPD

A Moment to Pause and Reflect

If you have come this far, you have already taken an important step.

You have chosen to understand your condition instead of fearing it.

That alone makes a difference.

COPD may be a chronic disease, but it is not the whole story of your life.

It is only one part of it.

A Shift in Perspective

At the beginning, most patients feel overwhelmed.

They think:

"Will my breathing keep getting worse?"

"Will I lose my independence?"

"What will happen to my future?"

These concerns are real.

But over time, something changes.

With understanding, patients begin to see COPD differently.

Not as something that completely defines them, but as something they can manage.

This shift in perspective is powerful.

From Fear to Control

Fear often comes from uncertainty.

When you do not understand what is happening, every symptom feels unpredictable.

But now, you know:

What COPD is

Why it happens

How to manage it

What to do when symptoms change

This knowledge gives you control.

And with control comes confidence.

Living with COPD, Not Against It

One of the most important lessons is this:

Do not fight your body. Work with it.

Some days will be better than others.

That is normal.

Living well with COPD means:

Listening to your body

Pacing your activities

Staying consistent with treatment

It is not about perfection.

It is about balance.

Small Wins, Big Impact

Improvement in COPD is often gradual.

It may not always be dramatic.

But small changes matter.

Walking a little farther

Feeling less breathless during routine tasks

Having fewer flare-ups

These are real achievements.

Over time, they add up to meaningful progress.

Staying Engaged with Life

COPD should not take you away from life.

Stay connected to:

Family

Friends

Activities you enjoy

Even simple moments:

A short walk

A conversation

Time with loved ones

bring value to your life.

Maintaining Independence

Independence is not about doing everything without help.

It is about maintaining control over your life.

With the right approach, you can:

Continue daily activities

Make your own decisions

Stay engaged

Accept help when needed, but stay involved.

The Importance of Routine

Routine creates stability.

Simple habits such as:

Taking medications on time

Staying active

Eating well

build a strong foundation.

Over time, these habits become part of your life.

Hope Is Realistic

Hope does not mean ignoring the disease.

It means recognizing what is still possible.

I have seen many patients:

Regain strength

Improve their activity level

Feel more confident

These outcomes are achievable.

A Final Patient Story

I remember a patient who once said to me:

“Doctor, I feel like my life is shrinking.”

We worked together on his treatment and daily routine.

Months later, he came back and said:

“I am not running, but I am living again.”

That is the goal.

Not perfection. Not cure.

But meaningful living.

What You Have Gained

By now, you understand:

What COPD is

How it develops

How to recognize symptoms

How to manage it with medications and lifestyle

How to prevent complications

How to live with confidence

This knowledge is powerful.

Your Role Moving Forward

Your doctor can guide you. Medications can help you.

But the most important role is yours.

Your daily actions determine:

How stable your condition remains

How active you can be

How you experience your life

This is your journey.

A Simple Way to Think About COPD

Let me leave you with a simple thought.

COPD may limit your breathing.

But it does not have to limit your life.

With:

Awareness

Consistency

Effort

Support

you can move forward with confidence.

Chapter Summary

COPD is a part of life, not the whole of it

Understanding replaces fear with control

Balance and consistency are key

Small improvements lead to meaningful progress

Staying engaged improves quality of life

Independence can be maintained

Routine builds stability

Hope is realistic and achievable

Action Plan for You

Stay consistent
Follow your treatment and routine

Focus on small progress
Every improvement matters

Stay connected
Engage with people and activities

Maintain a positive mindset
Balance realism with hope

Keep moving forward
One step at a time

Final Words

You are not defined by COPD.

You are defined by how you live, how you adapt, and how you move forward.

Take one step at a time. And keep going.

APPENDIX 1: Your Personal COPD Action Plan

My Daily Treatment Plan

Maintenance Inhalers (Daily Use):

____

____

Other Medications:

____

Oxygen Use (if prescribed):

____

____

My Rescue Plan (When Symptoms Worsen)

Rescue Inhaler Name:

____

How to Use (Dose and Frequency):

____

____

My Early Warning Signs

(Check what applies to you)

Increased breathlessness

More coughing than usual

Change in sputum color or amount

Chest tightness

Feeling more tired

Reduced ability to perform daily tasks

What I Will Do First

Use rescue inhaler as instructed

Rest and monitor symptoms

Follow my doctor's instructions

When I Will Call My Doctor

Symptoms not improving within 24–48 hours

Worsening breathlessness

Fever or signs of infection

Emergency – Seek Immediate Help If

Severe breathlessness

Unable to speak full sentences

Confusion or extreme fatigue

Bluish lips or fingertips

Important Contacts

Doctor Name and Phone:

____

Emergency Contact:

____

APPENDIX 2: Correct Inhaler Technique – Quick Reference

Basic Steps

Sit or stand upright

Exhale fully

Place inhaler correctly

Inhale slowly and deeply

Hold breath for 5–10 seconds

Exhale gently

Common Mistakes to Avoid

Not exhaling before use

Inhaling too quickly

Poor coordination

Not holding breath

Skipping doses

If using a steroid inhaler, rinse your mouth after use.

APPENDIX 3: COPD Medication Overview

Type	Purpose	When to Use	Common Side Effects
Rescue Inhaler	Quick relief	As needed	Tremor, fast heart rate
Long-Acting Inhaler	Maintain airflow	Daily	Dry mouth
Inhaled Steroid	Reduce inflammation	Selected patients	Throat irritation
Oral Medications	Reduce flare-ups	As prescribed	Varies

APPENDIX 4: Simple Exercise Plan

Walking Plan

Start with 5–10 minutes daily

Gradually increase to 20–30 minutes

Strength Exercises

Light weights or resistance bands

8–10 repetitions per session

2–3 times per week

Breathing Practice

Pursed-lip breathing daily

Use during activity

Important Tips

Start slowly

Stop if severe discomfort

Keep inhaler nearby

APPENDIX 5: Nutrition Guide

If You Are Underweight

Eat small, frequent meals

Focus on protein-rich foods

Include healthy calories

If You Are Overweight

Reduce portion size gradually

Focus on balanced meals

Combine with regular activity

General Tips

Eat slowly

Avoid heavy meals

Stay hydrated

APPENDIX 6: Emergency Information Sheet

Name: ______________________________

Diagnosis: COPD

Medications:

____

Allergies:

____

Doctor Contact:

____

Emergency Contact:

____

____

Thank You and

Please Review the Book

Thank you for taking the time to read this book. I sincerely hope it has helped you understand your health a little more clearly and has given you practical, everyday steps you can follow with confidence. If you found this book helpful, **I would truly appreciate it if you could leave a brief and honest review.** Even a few lines sharing your experience can make a meaningful difference. Your feedback helps other readers find reliable, trustworthy health information and supports them in making better decisions for themselves and their families.

Warm regards,

Dr Prabhat Das

Continue your Healthcare Journey

Good health is a journey, not a single step. It is not achieved in one day or with one book. That is why I created the **"Better Health with Dr Das Series",** with each book addressing a different common condition. If you would like easy, practical guidance on other everyday health concerns, you may wish to explore the rest of books in this series.

Books in this series:

Better Health starts Here: A Doctor's Guide to Staying Healthy After 40

A Doctor's Easy Guide to Understanding & Managing OBESITY

Doctor, What DIET Is Best for Me?

Doctor, Why Can't I Lose Weight? A Doctor's Guide to safe & Sustainable Weight Loss)

A Doctor's Easy Guide to GLP-1 for Obesity

A Doctor's Easy Guide to Understanding & Managing HIGH BLOOD PRESSURE

A Doctor's Guide to Living Well With DIABETES

A Doctor's Guide to Understanding & Managing THYROID DISEASES

A Doctor's Guide to Understanding & Managing HIGH CHOLESTEROL

A Doctor's Practical Guide to HEART HEALTH After 40: How to Protect Your Heart & Live Longer

A Doctor's Guide to Healing & Reversing FATTY LIVER DISEASE: Simple, Natural & Science-Based Steps to Reduce Liver Fat and Prevent Complications

Control Your ACID REFLUX, HEARTBURN & GERD: A Doctor's Practical Guide that Works

Live Comfortably with IRRITABLE BOWEL SYNDROME: A Doctor's Practical Guide to Understanding & Managing IBS

A Doctor's Practical Guide to Understanding & Managing GALLBLADDER STONES & OTHER PROBLEMS

Take Control of COPD: A Doctor's Practical Guide to Better Breathing

Living Better Life with ASTHMA: A Doctor's Practical Guide to Asthma Control

SLEEP APNEA & SNORING: A Doctor's Practical Guide to Better Sleep & Better Health

KIDNEY STONES: A Doctor's Practical Guide to Prevention & Care

Protect Your KIDNEYS: A Doctor's Practical Guide to Kidney Health & Prevention

PROSTATE HEALTH After 40: A Doctor's Practical Guide to Early Detection & Care

ARTHRITIS: A Doctor's Practical Guide to Pain Control & Mobility

A Doctor's Practical Guide to Fixing BACK PAIN Step by Step

A Doctor's Practical Guide to Understanding & Managing GOUT & URIC ACID and Preventing Complications

HEALTHY SKIN & COMMON SKIN PROBLEMS: A Doctor's Practical Guide to Skin Care

DEMENTIA & MEMORY LOSS: A Doctor's Practical Guide to Prevention & Management

Doctor, Why Am I TIRED All The Time? Fixing Fatigue & Getting Your Energy Back

www.ingramcontent.com/pod-product-compliance
Ingram Content Group UK Ltd.
Pitfield, Milton Keynes, MK11 3LW, UK
UKHW021959270726
14060UKWH00003B/597